Henri Rubinstein, M.D.

I0439324

# Are you spasmophilic ?

Spasmophilia or Chronic Tetany

Symptoms, predisposing factors, treatment
and prevention

## HENRI RUBINSTEIN, M.D.

Copyright © 2014 Henri Rubinstein, M.D.
All rights reserved.
ISBN : 1494886367
ISBN-13 : 9781494886363

DEDICATION

This book is dedicated to my patients.

CONTENTS

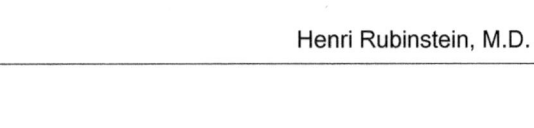
ACKNOWLEDGMENTS

The main scientific works refered to in this book are those of Doctors Duc, Durlach, Hioco, Klotz, Milhaud and Seyle.

# FOREWORD

Spasmophilia, also known as constitutional chronic tetany , is an extremely frequent disease in the daily practice of medicine.

Despite its being accepted in Europe by the general public, the media and advertisers, the attention paid to it by the medical profession would appear to be insufficient in relation to its real importance. For many physicians, spasmophilia is just a "fashion" disease, not a real one, and is attributed to stress, to the modern lifestyle, to present-day conditions of life - a disease brought about, in effect, by civilization. All this is true, but spasmophilia is far more than simply that.

It is an intriguing medical problem, because spasmophilia affects the organism in its physical, psychic and relational aspects,: a real demonstration of the subtle connection between organic pathology and the psychic disturbances. This somatic pathology leads to psychic disturbances which, in turn, maintain somatic pathology. This is the reason why a global approach is a better one for treating the disease.

We know of a large number of metabolic, biochemical, tissue, nervous and neurohormonal elements which affect this psychosomatic - or somatopsychic - circle. We know that spasmophilia is the common outcome of a number of objective disturbances- those disturbances are known, further research will shed light on what still remains obscure. But we have to explain the knowledge which has been acquired because of the very prominent role spasmophilia plays.

Principally, we have to give some hope to spasmophilics because they are patients who genuinely suffer. They have the right to understand their condition and to know that simple and effective medical therapy exists.

Because this book is intended for the general public, I will relate my own experiences, instead of expounding on scientific research on the subject of spasmophilia. My experience is based on 30,000 cases over a span of 30 years of practice in the realm of "functional exploration of the nervous system".

My work is based on a clinical and statistical analysis of those cases and their interpretation, on the medical literature on the subject and on contacts with the patients and their physicians.

This is a study not only of the disease itself, but also of its effect on the patients and on the physicians who treat them or rather fail to do so.

I

## SOME STORIES ABOUT SPASMOPHILICS

These summaries of clinical case histories are characteristic and have been chosen from amongst thousands. They help in understanding the practical problems of spasmophilia. It is useful to know and remember them before we begin a methodical description of the disease, its mechanisms and its treatments.

Mrs. B., 23 years old, is 3 months pregnant - first pregnancy. She complains of partial losses of consciousness. She and those close to her speak of bouts of fainting, and her gynecologist refers her to a cardiologist - "No organic cardiac pathology", says the cardiologist. Because the symptoms keep recurring, her blood sugar and blood calcium are tested - they are normal. The electroencephalograph is normal too. The diagnosis is "functional problems". Treated with sedatives, Mrs. B., complains throughout her pregnancy, of malaise and spasmodic vomiting. After the birth, she still feels very tired, and notices that her hair has split ends and her nails are cracked, and especially that her vision has become blurred. An ophthalmologist diagnoses a cataract - it is only at this stage that spasmophilia, which has been responsible for all her troubles, is diagnosed and treated, instead of this having been done a few months before. The cataract cannot be cured.

Mrs. H., 38 years old, real estate agent, is a dynamic active woman. She has been involved in a minor car accident. Her car was hit from behind. Mrs. H., does not suffer from loss of consciousness, there is no cranial trauma. X-rays of the head and neck are normal. During the subsequent weeks she suffers severe neck pains. She is exhausted, nervous and does not sleep well. She is afraid of going outside, cannot work anymore and becomes depressed. Her husband is worried, her physician advises her to consult a psychiatrist.

The psychiatrist diagnoses a premenopausal depression - chemotherapy does not bring any improvement, and Mrs. H. is hospitalized for 3 weeks in a clinic. She comes out a little better, but is still unable to get back to work. Only at this point does another physician discover that what has afflicted her is spasmophilia.

Mr. D., 35 years old, bank clerk, is worried about his professional future. He has become irascible, aggressive. He is tired, does not sleep well, and his work suffers. At nights he wakes up sweating, with chest pains. He gets up, has difficulty in breathing and goes back to bed. But the pain persists, compressing the chest. His wife panics and calls in a doctor. The electrocardiogram and the physical examination are normal. Mr. D., feels reassured and falls off to sleep. But the next morning he does not go to work. There is no more pain, but he is exhausted. He consults his general practitioner who sends him to a cardiologist. Here again, there is no pathology on examination, and "functional problems" are diagnosed. But Mr. D's health does not improve; his anxiety and tiredness increase. He goes back to work, but can no longer stand it. His nights are bad, with nightmares, and he wakes up tired. Only after several months is spasmophilia diagnosed, and treatment commenced.

Mrs. T., 35 years old, a housewife with three children, has always suffered from malaise ; at school, at the dentist, when giving a sample of blood. She faints frequently - she has always been of a nervous disposition. Now she has this tired feeling - her legs feel heavy. During the day she has to lie down because of a sudden feeling of weakness - somebody talked about "hypoglycemia", so she eats sugar as an antidote to her tiredness. Despite this, the tiredness persists and she gains weight. She consults a phlebologist, thinking she may have varicose veins because of her heavy legs. The phlebologist finds no varicose veins but diagnoses spasmophilia, confirmed by further examinations.

Miss. S., 30 years old, a spinster, is a bookkeeper and has always suffered from headaches. A month ago she began complaining of terrible migraines ; she has to stay in bed, keeps vomiting, and cannot stand light anymore. Miss. S., fears a brain tumor. Her physician finds no abnormalities and further examinations are negative. The treatment she gets is not very effective. At this point, the doctor discovers that her headaches started after she had been on diet. {Miss S., had wanted to lose a few kilos before the summer.) Then it dawns on him that it might be spasmophilia.

Mr. K., 57 years old, a watchman in a factory. He has been in the colonies and he is convinced that he picked up amoebae there ; anyway he suffers from abdominal pains. He feels swollen and distended, and suffers from aerophagie. He goes from diarrhea to constipation. He is also very tired and especially depressed on account of his wife having left him. He has visited a number of gastroenterologists and was also hospitalized for further observations, but no signs of amoeba were detected in his stools. His abdominal pains still disturb him. This has been going for years and Mr. K-, has been going from one doctor to another. Here again, spasmophilia will eventually be diagnosed.

The young Michael D-, 10 years old, is a healthy child, a little on the noisy side. From the beginning of the school year, he has not been doing very well, and is continually tired. At home he does not eat well, and sleeps a lot. He has difficulty in waking each morning. All these little troubles make his mother very anxious and she consults a pediatrician. He finds no abnormalities and prescribes a tonic. For two or three months there is no improvement, and his schoolwork gets steadily worse. The child complains of headaches. Again the pediatrician is consulted. He calls for on an electroencephalograph, which gives rise to a suspicion of spasmophilia, which is later confirmed.

Mrs. T., 43 years old, a nurse, suffers from endometriosis (a disease of the uterus, hormonal in origin, characterized by a thickening of the internal wall of this organ). After her husband's death, she complains of considerable uterine bleeding. This loss of blood is so profuse that she has to be hospitalized. All examinations are negative, and the haemostatic treatment (the object of which is to stop the bleeding) is ineffective. Mrs. T., is still bleeding. She has to receive several blood transfusions. Her general health is badly affected and she becomes terribly tired. The diagnosis of spasmophilia is made only several months afterwards. The treatment for spasmophilia stops the bleeding and the patient is cured.

What is this mysterious illness which affects patients and confuses physicians ?

# WHAT IS SPASMOPHILIA ?

Spasmophilia is a very common disease which afflicts about seven to eight million French people. It is responsible for very a wide range of symptoms, such as tiredness, muscular cramps, nervous breakdowns, anxiety and insomnia, and is a veritable plague to those who endure this daily torment.

In spite of the fact that a large part of the population suffers from such problems, very few know anything about it. For the general public, as well as for many physicians, the origin of these symptoms is attributed in a hazy sort of way to the present day pace of life, to stress, or psychiatric difficulties. This confusion no longer applies today because we know that spasmophilia is an authentic disease which can be defined by accurate chemical, physiological and biological criteria. The knowledge of such criteria makes it possible to define the illness, to diagnose it and to treat it.

Spasmophilia is, on the one hand, paraphysiological, and on the other, pathological ; characterized by an excessive and persistent neuromuscular stimulation. This state is responsible for several symptoms which are detailed below. There is no other medical explanation or any specific macrolesions as a source for symptoms behind this neuromuscular overstimulation.

The characteristic signs which determine the diagnosis are at three levels.

1°/ Clinical - In other words: the symptoms that the patient complains of, additional symptoms that the patient evokes in the interview, and objective signs at the examination.
2°/ Electrophysiological - principally the electromyogram.
3°/ Biological : the measurement of certain ions in the organism - in the blood or urine.

Only when we begin to understand the principal mechanism which plays a part in the production of symptoms of spasmophilia, can we affirm this distinct pathological entity. In other words, it is a microlesional organic disease with metabolic, biochemical and neurohormonal elements.

The symptoms of spasmophilia are neither an ineluctable consequence of modern life, nor the masks of an hysterical neurosis. They are manifestations of a pathological state that we have to recognize and treat.

Spasmophilia is a very frequent disease, pathological on the. one hand, and paraphysiological on the other. This brings us immediately to the fact that there are two patterns to the disease :

Latent spasmophilia - having epidemiological implications among the population. Patients have certain symptoms that are not disturbing or important enough to bring them to a physician's consulting room. In many cases they are not even aware of them. This is why one can be a spasmophilic and not even know about it. But this a vulnerable situation. Some trigger - we will see what these are and how we are exposed to them - some sort of spark will disturb this delicate equilibrium and latent spasmophilia will turn into decompensated spasmophilia.

Decompensated spasmophilia is a genuine disease, a daily torment, sometimes a dramatic one. The exacerbation of symptoms, their permanence, and their disabling nature, are what bring the patient to the physician.

The term "spasmophilia" has its origin in Greek and literally means "affinity for spasms". It explains the duality of the disease by using the term "affinity", in other words, predisposition and propensity. This term is much better that the older one : "tetany", sometimes still in use. "Tetany" was classicaly associated with an insufficient secretion of the parathyroid glands - this is a long way from the present pathogenic concept of the disease. We will see later in this treatise that in a particular manifestation, the use of the term "tetany crisis" is justified. More than that, the term "spasmophilia" accentuates the factor of spasm, in other words, the muscular contraction. This contraction can affect all the muscles in the body : the striated voluntary muscles, as well as the smooth involuntary muscles. The contraction is, effectively, the focal point in the symptoms of spasmophilia. We will see how the neuromuscular overstimulation is responsible for this. One can easily understand that spasms explain many other symptoms, such as anxiety or insomnia, which are not satisfactorily described by the term given to the disease.

Historically, spasmophilia was first recognized in France ; in fact, in 1852, Lucien Corvisart, a descendant of Napoleon's doctor, devoted his thesis to the contraction of extremities, something he called "tetania". Trousseau, ten years later in 1862, in a famous lecture described the "rheumatic" contraction of nursing mothers in a most masterful fashion {he emphasized the fact that breast feeding is a trigger for predisposition to spasmophilia.

In 1876, Chvostek, a Hungarian physician, described the symptom of percussion on the facial nerve. This has been named after him. It is one of the major clinical signs in the physical examination of a spasmophilic.

Professors Turpin and Lefebvre introduced the practice of electromyograms in 1943. It enables the isolation of the electro-physiological elements of the disease.

In 1950, Professors Justin-Besancon and Klotz gave the term spasmophilia to the disease. Only recently has the disease been recognized by the Anglo-Saxon medical world. Raisen described it in the United States in terms of being a "hyperventilation syndrome". We will examine this last term which accentuates the respiratory problems which spark off the symptoms of spasmophilia.

# WHO IS SPASMOPHILIC ?

Spasmophilia is a highly prevalent disease. In its latent and decompensated forms it affects between 12 and 20 percent of the French population, about 6 to 10 million people, and probably a similar percentage in all developed countries.

The figure of 14 percent is generally accepted for France, which entails more than seven and a half million. Such a figure indicates that the medical problem is also truly a social problem at several levels :

- Financially for the community ; medical costs, the cost for sick leave in work-hours lost, and often-unnecessary hospitalization.

- In its general impact on the population ; so many patients, fatigued, anxious, depressed, fragile, must be detrimental to the stability of the country.

- In respect of measures of prevention as we shall see, which are imperative and which can only be decided on by the Health Ministry.

Spasmophilia may be a social problem, but it is also a question of personal genetic make up. A disease which is so widespread in the population must have a hereditary base. We will see that the mechanisms of spasmophilia, over and above the various metabolic and deficiency elements, concern the permeability of the cellular membranes. These disturbances of the cellular membrane permeability are probably part of the genetic heritage of certain individuals and one could be spasmophilic on the same basis as one has blue eyes. More exactly, a part of the population has a spasmophilic terrain, a latent spasmophilia that could decompensate itself.

Spasmophilia reaches about as many men as women, and even though generally a predominance of women over men is recorded {3 to 4 women to 1 man), this could be due to the socio-cultural fact that women generally consult physicians more often than men, and particularly for this type of disturbance.

In the American statistics covering the syndrome of hyperventilation, the incidence of sex appears negligible, and in any case, there is no preponderance of women in surveys involving large numbers.

One can be spasmophilic at all ages, but predominance is noted between puberty and the fifties. Nevertheless, there are spasmophilics among children, even newborn, and likewise in elderly people. Since it concerns a latent disease which decompensates under the effect of external circumstances, as we shall see, it is understandable that one is more exposed to the factors of decompensation at the active stages of life rather than at the early and late stages.

There do not seem to be any special ethnical factors in spasmophilics, but it is certain that the most severe and explosive forms very often attack people not indigenous to the population. Forms of spasmophilia in which the symptoms reach maximum intensity are often found in people coming from areas overseas (Antilles, the Reunion), who come to work in France. The radical change in life and feeding habits may constitute a primary triggering factor, in these cases.

Spasmophilia is to be found in all social classes and is certainly not a "class illness". Workers, clerks, middle and top managerial staff, company executives, artists, professional people, physicians and others, present the same symptoms which makes all of them distressed. The level of education does not seem to play a role and the description of the disturbances is surprisingly similar among the simple-minded as among the most educated. At most, among the latter, there is a greater descriptive variety, but with no major difference. Habitat plays no preponderent influence. There are as many spasmophilics in rural areas as in the towns.

This single fact that individuals of different milieus, culture and social levels, present so remarkably the same symptoms, is further proof that the matter is not a cultural discourse or a way to put a name on something unknown, but constitutes a deep disturbance, constitutional and metabolic. Many people have at one time or another presented pathological manifestations for which their physician could not find a clear-cut organic cause. These pathological manifestations have then been stowed away under terms such as "neurovegetative dystonia", "sympathetic irregularity", "functional pathology", or "neurotonic". It is highly probable that these terms concern an unrecognized spasmophilia.

## ARE YOU SPASMOPHILIC ?

The description of spasmophilia symptoms covers a vast area of medical pathology and it is easy to understand that those who are afflicted consult with general practitioners or various specialists. It is without doubt impossible to set up an exhaustive list of all the symptoms of spasmophilia, so great is the polymorphism of the disease. It is at times tempting, in regard to authenticated spasmophilics, to link certain aberrant symptoms to spasmophilia. This temptation should be put aside, and this is precisely the task of the physician. His training should allow him to distinguish between what is most likely to be related to spasmophilia and what concerns some other etiology. Statistical arguments and frequency factors will comprise the best guides of medical practice to allow the linking of a given symptom to this disease.

The symptoms that I am about to describe are therefore those that one comes across in numerous patients. As in every illness, there are general symptoms, namely those which pertain to the entire organism, and localized symptoms, those that apply to a particular system. This way of approaching the description of the symptoms of the disease should be considered as an introduction which applies somewhat artificial categories for the clarity of the outline. It corresponds to the usual categories in medicine but it must not be forgotten that neuromuscular stimulation relates to physiological structures which exist in the entire organism and in all the organs.

- The general symptoms : these are dominated by fatigue (asthenia) in more than 90 percent of the cases, and this destructively characteristic fatigue occurs mainly in the mornings. Spasmophilics wake up tired ; their night's rest, good or bad, has done them no good. This fatigue tends to taper off during the day but at the same time there will be a severe drop-off in energy with feelings of total prostration. Sometimes these episodes of severe fatigue are present without morning asthenia.

Among other general symptoms are disturbances in thermal regulation : chilliness and/or sudden flushes, as well as disturbances in eating habits; anorexia or bulimia, the source of weight loss or gain.

Psychic signs can also be considered as part of the general symptoms since they control the relationships and the emotional life of the patient.

These psychic symptoms may be of varying importance from simple nervousness to emotivity accompanied by outbursts of temper, and even attacks of anxiety. Frequent anger, attacks of laughter or tears is often part of the minimal symptoms of spasmophilia. Anxiety is virtually constant. It can range from apprehension, to a tendency to worry, a tendency to make mountains out of molehills to states of truly disabling anxiety. This disabling anxiety is more prevalent among spasmophilics ; it cramps them in their daily life, in their relationships and in their work. The anxiety manifests itself in the shape of a sensation of a "ball in the throat", the impression of suffocating, of imminent death. There are repeated bouts of cold sweats, attacks of tears or trembling. More severely, the anxiety makes it impossible to carry out the most simple of acts; great difficulty in getting up, trepidation in going out, fear of crowds, of going into large shops, fear of large open spaces (agoraphobia) or even fear of taking an elevator or being closed-in (claustrophobia).

The anxiety, we shall see, is a symptom proper to spasmophilia, and is linked to neuro-hormonal disturbances. This anxiety is also maintained and increased by other symptoms of the disease : the sensation of suffocating provokes fear, as doe's pain in the region of the heart. The fear of having a malaise and fainting, keeps the patient at home. Anxiety explains the sadness of the spasmophilics, their drawn features, and their occasionally dejected and dismal appearance.

The anxiety of spasmophilics is often complicated by depressive states, in which the patients have no interest in life, are "down in the dumps" and abandon all relational activity. Disturbances of sleep are extremely common and persistent, the most frequent insomnia occuring during the latter part of the night : the patient wakes up at two or three in the morning and cannot go back to sleep. If he does, he has terrifying nightmares, often dreaming that he is falling. Sometimes he tosses in bed for hours and finally falls asleep again in the early morning. This insomnia adds to the exhaustion of patients who are already fatigued and with a propensity for being tired out.

The general symptoms and psychic signs of spasmophilia, that is, mainly fatigue, anxiety and insomnia, are the most instructive, because they are often the least understood and the most painful to the patients. These symptoms make their lives distressing, even unbearable, making them suffer and cut them off from the world of the healthy. Their consequences are also the most dramatic for they lead to recourse to anti-anxiety and antidepressant chemotherapy, even to psychiatric treatment, always ineffective and dangerous for spasmophilics.

Localized symptoms concern more particularly various physiological structures or groups of organs ; they are :

a) The signs of neuromuscular overstimulation proper :

- muscular cramps ;
- tingling (paresthesias) in the hands and feet ;
- tingling in the throat (pharyngeal paresthesia) ;
- myoclonias (involuntary muscular twitching) ;
- palpebral clonias (eyelids that jump or quiver) ;
- pain in the spinal column at the level of the cervical, the thoracic or the lumbar region (without involving arthritic lesions and which are due to a contraction of the paravertebral muscles).

b) Vasomotor signs, i.e., those linked to spasms of the blood vessels:

- headaches (cephaleas) which can be diverse : all over the head or localized, such as retro-orbital, frontal, and true migraines localized at one side of the head. They can be permanent or occur as attacks;

- lipothymias, brief loss of consciousness preceded by an intense feeling of being unwell, often with thoracic oppression, tingling of the fingers and the mouth ; spasmophilics faint easily but these malaises may not go as far as a complete loss of consciousness.

There are also sensations of dizziness and vertigo, sensations of hazy and blurred vision, signs of orthostatic hypotension {dizziness resulting from a sudden change of position), vasomotor disturbances of the extremities from a banal chill to the Raynaud syndrome (fingers which turn white and are insensitive to cold).

c) Visceral signs that concern deep organs, those that reproduce the symptoms spoken of under neurovegetative dystonia: they can be connected with :

- the cardiovascular system: palpitations, tachycardia, thoracic pain and oppression ;

- the digestive system: various digestive disturbances, pseudogastric, pseudobiliary, pseudocolitic, constipation ;

- the respiratory system : pseudo-asthmatic respiratory oppression, sensation of a tightening of the larynx, the well-known "ball in the throat" so often mentioned by the patients.

d) Symptoms concerning the phaneras, that is, fingernails soft and doubled, fragile and brittle hair, frequent and seriously decayed teeth, opacity of the crystalline lens which can lead to a cataract, serious and unusual in young patients, and corresponding to specific ophthalmologic criteria (cataract in the posterior capsule).

e) Signs that relate to the genital area:

in women, spontaneous abortions, pelvic pain, vaginismus and frigidity; in men, premature ejaculation, loss of sperm, impotence.

f) Attacks of tetany itself are often extremely characteristic, but occur relatively infrequently.

These are violent painful attacks of contraction, starting at the extremities and extending to the entire body. The hand goes into hyperextension, the palm becomes hollow, the extended fingers overlap into the "midwife's hand". The foot goes into extension and twists around. The group of contractions of hands and feet is called carpopedal spasm. In the face, the muscle contractions deform the mouth so that it looks like the snout of a carp. Extending to the paravertebral, the contraction arches the body.

Many spasmophilics have never had an attack of tetany and may never have one. It is highly dramatic and spectacular for the patient and those close to him, but not really dangerous. It has the advantage of making the diagnosis of spasmophilia obvious, even to an inexperienced physician, and thus avoids many mistaken diagnoses.

These attacks of tetany, particularly if they come at the beginning of the illness, act as an alarm signal for the patient, those close to him and his physician, and even if the spasmophilia is not necessarily better treated, at least the patient is aware of the nature of his disturbances.

Finally it should be noted that numerous signs of spasmophilia are found in ailments still poorly understood, such as: allergies, essential arterial hypertension in young people, idiopathic cyclic edemas (without precise cause); functional hypoglycemia, thyroid dysfunction. These very diverse malaises have in common their functional character, and it is likely but not yet certain that nervous and muscular overstimulation plays a role in the appearance of these diseases.

This long list of symptoms is not of course present in all spasmophilics but usually patients have at least about ten of the symptoms described above, of which the most important are often fatigue, malaises, headaches, anxiety, muscular fatigue, etc.

There is also what is referred to as "multisymptomatic" spasmophilia. It is these multisymptomatic forms which are prevalent amongst young adults and are most frequently seen by general practitioners. However, there are also many misleading forms with very few symptoms ("paucisymptomatic"). This applies to patients all of whose symptoms are concentrated within a single system and who consult with the specialists; the gastroenterologists for digestive disturbances, cardiologists for palpitations and thoracic pain, the ear, nose and throat specialists, for vertigo and buzzing in the ears, rheumatologists for vertebral pain and often neuro-psychiatrists for insomnia, anxiety and depressive states.

# WHEN LATENT SPASMOPHILIA IS DECOMPENSATED

As I have outlined, spasmophilia is latent at first ; that is to say, a large proportion of the population manifests paraphysiological conditions of excessive neuromuscular stimulation, the symptoms being those described above, but to a certain extent, spasmophilics have little or no awareness of their condition. They are to be found at the extremes of those symptoms which can appear as simple nervousness. But they are in a delicate balance and a simple surge can make them verge into spasmophilia, an illness that will show up markedly. The term for this is "decompensation". This concept of decompensation is what explains the interest in knowing about and being able to diagnose latent spasmophilia. For, though it is often possible to treat decompensated spasmophilia, it is far better to seek to prevent it, all the more so because neuromuscular overstimulation is something very common in the population and as such there are innumerable situations which can bring on decompensation.

Every spasmophilic faces the threat of decompensation of his illness. It must be realized that if there seems at the present time to be a rise in the number of spasmophilics, it is not because their number has multiplied, but because the factors which cause decompensation are infinitely more numerous and it is somewhat rare not to encounter one or more during a lifetime. I would likewise mention at this point (but will develop the idea later) that the modern diet, especially over refined foodstuffs, is the cause for various deficiencies, particularly of magnesium, something which was not the case in the past.

The group of decompensatory factors can be put under the heading of "stress", that is to say, aggression against the body. These aggressions can be physical or emotional in a wide sense. But a factor of decompensation is found in every spasmophilic and the exact time this started is capable of being assessed quite clearly. It is up to the physician to find the cause that triggered the surge of spasmophilia if the patient himself is unable to pinpoint it.

Genuine overwork is the most frequent triggering factor; it might be tied up with one professional activity or another, brief and intense on the one hand, or, of a prolonged nature on the other. Almost equally prevalent are recent psychological difficulties : family or professional conflicts and sexual problems. There are also medicinal factors (prolonged ingestion of laxatives or diuretics) ; and illness, chronic infection or recent viral infection. Reducing diets are often the cause of a surge of spasmophilia. Other factors of decompensation are traffic accidents, traumas, mourning, and surgery.

There are decompensation factors that apply specifically to women: pregnancy, breast-feeding, miscarriage, hysterectomy, gynecological infection and the ingestion of contraceptives ("the pill"). Seasonable increases in autumn and spring and a premenstrual increase among young women have also been noted.

Among contributing factors are family antecedents and a psychological disposition marked by tendency toward anxiety or obsessions, rather banal until the occurrence of the symptoms, but whose role then appears evident in contributing to and aggravating the symptoms.

When the spasmophilia is decompensated the patient becomes ill. I insist on a precise determination of the inception of the troubles which is a remarkably consistent feature noted in the observation of spasmophilics. What is frequently heard is "I don't feel well since I had that automobile accident," or "I am tired out and my legs hurt since my confinement," or even "since my son passed his bachelors exams after working so hard and succeeding, he is perpetually tired and listless."

All these patients are conscious that their condition has changed, that something has happened, that something is "unsettled". They all express the will to get back to their former condition and to recover their equilibrium. We will see that this precise knowledge as to the start of their symptoms and this wish to find a solution is one of the differences between spasmophilics and neurotics.

# THE DAILY LIFE OF SPASMOPHILICS

Spasmophilia is an illness which, without being dangerous or life threatening, is extremely painful. The symptoms of fatigue, anxiety, insomnia, are very trying in daily life and present problems in human relationships that can become quite dramatic. These fatigued and anxious patients find it hard to carry out their everyday chores ; and their family life shows the effects : family quarrels, separations and divorces are frequent. Their professional activity is often badly affected due to problems brought on by their being absent from work. Their anxiety and the difficulty they find in being active, have consequences which affect the progress of their career. They are dispirited on account of fatigue and anxiety. Contact with them is often unpleasant. They hesitate to leave their home for fear of malaise and tend to live the life of a recluse.

The life of spasmophilics is often a daily torment; they feel an early morning anxiety ; the malaise of going to work, the impression of being short of air, of suffocating, heavy arms, tense and painful muscles. Exhausted at their work, they come home irritable and aggressive, or as opposed to that, dejected, interested in nothing. Their faces often show sadness as well as despair, giving an impression of being condemned with no possibility of ever getting free.

If their physician is not acquainted with spasmophilia and decides that they are not ill or that they are just "nervous" (the implication being that everything is imaginary), they feel misunderstood and neglected and all the more so when those close to them blame them, frequently severely, for their condition. This makes them feel bitter and deepens their anxiety and depression still further.

Spasmophilics know they are ill, they suffer from their malaise, they suffer from their anxiety, they suffer from their lack of ability to adapt to daily life and they regret what is happening to them and want to get back to a normal existence. That, I repeat, is the great difference between neurotics, who take delight in their situation and whose illness constitutes a reason to go on living, and spasmophilics whose illness is what prevents them from enjoying life.

This difference is fundamental and I will come back to the problems of neurosis, because to many psychiatrists spasmophilia is simply a neurosis - an attitude which leads to an overconsumption of inefficient and dangerous chemotherapies. The enormous consumption of anti-anxiety drugs, anti-depressants and sleeping pills, gives an idea as to the truth of this viewpoint, with 5 to 10 million Frenchmen being turned into psychiatric cases.

Fortunately some physicians, and not the least of them, know that spasmophilia is an illness, and before studying the clinical observations and the treatment, they have tried to understand the mechanisms ; that will be the subject for the next chapter.

# THE MECHANISM OF SPASMOPHILIA

The mechanism of spasmophilia has not yet been entirely cleared up but a certain number of processes have been shown to intervene in the creation of symptoms of neuromuscular overstimulation and those of psychic symptoms. The main factors, as well as their roles in the creation of this illness, are likewise known. Similarly, different structures of the body are brought into play by spasmophilia. They are the striated muscles (voluntary muscles), the central nervous system, the peripheral nervous system, the autonomous nervous system, the neuromuscular junctions, and finally, various hormones and the endocrine glands that secrete them.

We will see that spasmophilia brings about a true pathology of microlesions ; in other words, at its origin, there exist small but authentic lesions of numerous organs and constituents of the human body. These microlesions are qualitatively different from much larger lesions that are observed in classic organic pathology. The difference is uniquely quantitative but the substratum of the lesion is organic as well, for the functional difficulties of the organs are linked to microlesions which are becoming progressively better known. This is what enables us to say that the functional pathology is organic.

To understand what spasmophilia is, one must schematically set up an axis that includes :
- the conscious brain;
- the unconscious brain;
- the sensory and motor nervous system pathways;
- the autonomous system nerve pathways;
- the hormonal ducts;
- the smooth musculature
- the striated musculature.

In this diagram, spasmophilia occurs at the level of neuromuscular excitability, and the original trouble is a disturbance of this neuromuscular stimulation. All living cells have the possibility of contracting, more especially the nerve and muscle cells. The means of this contraction are the positive ions (bodies charged with positive electricity present in the cells and around the cells), sodium, potassium, calcium, magnesium and hydrogen. The passage of these ions in one or other direction across the cell membrane will determine the excitability of these cells. This passage is both autonomous and controlled by various hormones. The excitability of the nerve and muscle cells depends therefore on the permeability of the cellular membrane (the membrane which encloses every cell) and on the passage of ions through this membrane.

The excitability of the cells varies according to the Loeb equation:

$$\frac{\text{SODIUM + POTASSIUM}}{\text{MAGNESIUM + CALCIUM + HYDROGENE}} \qquad \frac{(Na^+ + K^+)}{(H^+ + Mg^{2+} + Ca^{2+})}$$

Each time that this ratio increases, the excitability steps up. It is therefore easily understood that an increase of this ratio creates an increase of neuromuscular stimulation. It thus follows that the symptoms of spasmophilia can be due to a reduction in the ions present in the lower part of this ratio. In particular, a hyperexcitability can be triggered by a lowering of ionized calcium, by the reduction of ionized magnesium, and by the reduction of hydrogenated ions. These then are the elements of the ionic theory of spasmophilia.

The ionic theory introduces a primary ionic trouble, either by lack of supply, or by faulty regulation.

It has been shown, for example, that there is a lack of magnesium in the food supply; the overall quantity in the body of magnesium is 22 to 28 grams and the daily requirements are evaluated at 7 to 10 milligrams per kilo body weight. It has been determined that the daily food ration contains little more than 4 milligrams of magnesium per kilo of body weight. The reasons for this deficit in magnesium are numerous and will be detailed later.

The existence of a chronic lack in the supply of magnesium is the basis of the "magnesium theory" for spasmophilia. For those who hold to this hypothesis spasmophilia is the primary form of a deficit in magnesium.

There is likewise the possibility of trouble in the supply of calcium. The amount of calcium in the body is high. This calcium is mainly fixed in the bones and the level of calcium in the blood of spasmophilics is always within the normal range. However, by using radioactive calcium measurements, it has been proved that the calcium pool is reduced in these patients and in particular the level of intracellular calcium is lowered. Me will see that the maintenance of a normal level of blood calcium in the body is obtained by draining the calcium from the bones which makes them weaker (osteoporosis).

The reduction of hydrogen ions is the mechanism which underlies the Anglo-Saxon concept of spasmophilia, called in the U.S.A. the syndrome of chronic hyperventilation ; indeed a chronic hyperventilation brings on a respiratory alkalosis, and therefore a reduction in H ions. The reduction of H ions in the Loeb formula thus produces a hyperexcitability.

To the ionic theories can be added the hypothesis of the existence in spasmophilia of a reduction of phosphorus, the role of which is to maintain calcium and magnesium in the cells; a lack of phosphorus would bring on a leakage of intracellular calcium and magnesium.

Finally, the permeability of the cellular membrane is modified in spasmophilics. This is without doubt the constitutional factor proper to this disease. The vitamin D that intervenes to promote the intracellular passage of calcium and magnesium intervenes in spasmophilics to reduce the ionic losses of these cells.

But the ionic disturbances, whatever their importance, do not suffice to explain the mechanisms of spasmophilia. Neuromuscular excitability depends, moreover, on the neuro-mediators and the neuro-modulators, among them adrenalin.

Adrenalin is secreted at the level of the medullo-adrenal gland and at the level of the fiber terminals of the sympathetic nervous system (autonomous nervous system) where it is the natural agent for the transmission of nervous impulses. Adrenalin is secreted in excess in the case of spasmophilics, something that has been proven by numerous biological measurements. However, it is likewise known that against all stress - that is, all external aggression in the widest sense - the body reacts by a discharge of adrenalin, then by a permanent increase in the adrenalin secretion. Psychological factors, in particular in states of anxiety, play a role in the liberation of adrenalin from the medullo-adrenal gland by acting on the centers of emotion which are located in the limbic brain. In addition, the alkalosis itself, that is the reduction of H ions increases the production of adrenalin due to a modification in the oxygenation of the nervous tissues.

We have seen the determinant decompensating role of all aggression and all stress in spasmophilics. Adrenalin increases excitability, consequently the massive secretion of adrenalin provokes an overstimulation and can decompensate the spasmophilia. But when overstimulation is present, adrenalin increases anxiety and creates fatiguing symptoms (insomnia, cramps) and anxiety symptoms (palpitations, malaises) which then increase the secretion of adrenalin. This sets up a vicious circle where the symptoms add to the causes and the causes add to the symptoms.

This first vicious circle (the hyperexcitability which increases the secretion of adrenalin which in turn increases the hyperexcitability) is not the only one in question, because adrenalin has the physiological effect of masking the sensation of fatigue. But masking the sensation of fatigue is done at the price of an increase in the consumption of energy, an increase in muscular tension, and finally, at the price of an excitation injurious to sleep. These three factors are in themselves the deep causes of fatigue in spasmophilics. These three factors momentarily mask the fatigue, but it is only a camouflage of what constitutes a true flight forward. This second vicious circle (adrenalin combats fatigue by methods which tire out the system and increase the production of adrenalin) is not the last, for most probably a third exists: the ionic disturbances themselves act at the level of the brain on the regulation of the endocrine mechanisms which are improperly excited and disturbed. Overstimulation brings on faulty regulation of the endocrine system which keeps up this hyperexcitability.

Spasmophilia then truly is a condition of neuromuscular hyperexcitability, decompensated by stress of variable nature. We have just seen that there are vicious circles which maintain and perpetuate the spasmophilia. This self-maintenance continues from the time when the vicious circles producing the symptoms - the metabolic and endocrine disturbances have taken hold - even if one or more of the trigger factors have disappeared.

Spasmophilia is an illness in which all the disturbances feed on themselves.

Professor Duc has assembled the main factors identified in spasmophilia in the drawing below :

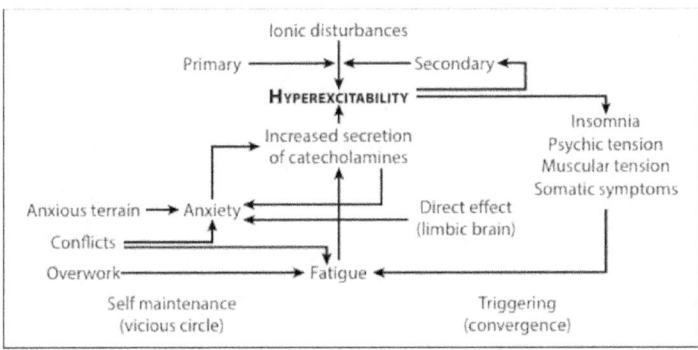

Before closing this chapter, I insist on the fact that the mode of production of the symptoms of spasmophilia is organic. It concerns the transmission of information in a wide sense by an excited neuron. This neuron has been excited by a pathological stimulus or by a repetition of pathological stimuli. The symptoms are not cerebral creations, which are more or less unconscious : when a spasmophilic suffers he really does suffer in the manner I have outlined above.

# II

## SPASMOPHILIA AND GENERAL CONDITION

The comprehension of the general mechanisms of spasmophilia calls for understanding the extreme diversity of the manifestations of this disease. However, the impact on the general condition is of prime importance and before considering the symptoms of spasmophilia, system by system, it would be right to dwell on the repercussion of neuro-muscular overstimulation on the body as a whole ; that is, the general symptoms of the disease.

The general condition is understood here in a wide sense, which signifies the sensation of well-being and equilibrium of the individual as well as the physical condition of his body, the harmony of its forms and features, its beauty, its energy, its activities.

The main general symptoms of spasmophilia are: fatigue, which may take various different forms (morning fatigue, an abnormal tendency to be fatigued), the effect on the body which could be disturbances of weight (obesity or emaciation) but also modifications of the face, drawn features, bags under the eyes; disturbances in the mechanisms of thermal regulation, in particular certain extended feverish states without apparent explanation; finally disturbances in sleep, insomnia, nightmares or on the contrary, hypersomnia.

Fatigue is one of the principle symptoms of spasmophilia, this fatigue being intense and absolutely characteristic, for it is found in at least 90 percent of cases. It is a morning fatigue: always present on awakening, even after a good night's sleep. At times it is so pronounced that the patient has to remain in bed. This fatigue often goes far back in time, with no explanation for it; it is part of the daily life of these patients who feel that this is their fate.

These perpetually fatigued patients have few interests ; for them everything calls for an effort, at times insuperable. Although the morning fatigue is often present, another form of fatigue is also frequent in spasmophilics : the feeling of being "fagged out", that is the brutal feeling of exhaustion which comes on during the day, either during the afternoon or after meals. Up to then activity has been normal, when suddenly the patient feels exhausted, empty ; he has to break off what he has been doing, and sit down and rest.

He can sustain no physical effort; he is totally worn out. It could be an attack of weakness or even an abnormal tiredness - difficulty in carrying a valise, the inability to take a long walk.

The different forms of fatigue and exhaustion are part of the spasmophilic's daily life. They are aware that they can run up against fatigue at any time, no matter what they do. Often fatigue makes them forego their activities. They hesitate to leave their home knowing that their exhaustion will prevent them from enjoying what they do. Fatigue is at the center of these patients' lives and this symptom is so common, so habitual, that they feel it is part of their personality. Physicians confronted with this manifestation of fatigue are almost always powerless if they don't happen to consider spasmophilia. Indeed, medicaments for stimulation, for "defatiguing" or for fortifying, so habitually prescribed, only aggravate matters by boosting these patients up and increasing their hyperexcitability.

The overall repercussion on the body is part of the general symptoms which are characteristic of spasmophilia. More often than not these are disturbances in weight : obesity, in which bulimia or excess of food doubtless have a role, but many cases of overweight appear in subjects who do not overeat.

The delicate disturbances in metabolism then come to the fore and very often spasmophilia is a constituent factor. Anorexia, which brings on emaciation, and abnormal underweight are equally prevalent among spasmophilics. Besides obesity and blatant underweight, the faces of spasmophilics have a characteristic appearance: bags under the eyes from fatigue and insomnia can be a daily problem. Drawn features, deep wrinkles that age the person prematurely, are caused by the permanent muscular tension which justifiably distresses these patients. A balanced body is the best sign of beauty, while spasmophilia is one of the principal causes of physical and psychological maladjustment.

The disturbances in thermal regulation bring us back to the pathology proper. We often observe low-grade fever in spasmophilics - (38 to 38.5 degrees) for which there is no explanation. The patients have seen many physicians ; all of the diagnostic investigations, other than those concerning spasmophilia, have turned out to be negative and remain negative and it is then justifiable to believe that a deep disturbance of the mechanisms of thermal homeostasis linked to neuromuscular stimulation is involved.

Disturbances in sleep are most prominent amongst spasmophilics. Classically this entails insomnia during the second part of the night, which aggravates the fatigue and engenders anxiety and a state of depression. The account of sleep disturbances, so characteristic of the general condition of spasmophilics, will be developed further when we come to discuss the effect this illness has on the psyche.

## SPASMOPHILIA AND CARDIO-VASCULAR DISEASES

We have seen that the localization of spasmophilic symptoms on the heart and blood vessels is extremely frequent, producing palpitations, acceleration of the heart rhythm (tachycardia), sensations of pain and thoracic oppression, and likewise vascular disturbances of the extremities by arterial spasm (bloodless fingers).

The mechanism for the production of these symptoms can be explained by muscular spasms: either of the voluntary striated musculature or of the involuntary smooth musculature which is found inside the blood vessels. The secretion of adrenalin which we have noted increases in spasmophilia, intervenes likewise by its own role of acceleration of the cardiac rhythm and vasoconstriction.

Finally, a third mechanism - hyperventilation - intervenes, creating a respiratory alkalosis (that is an increase of the blood PH factor) ; this respiratory alkalosis has likewise a vasoconstrictor effect at the arterial level.

Vascular spasms explain the chest pains which may be acute and are often described as a thrust of flame or knife. In addition, the spasms, if they touch the coronary arteries (arteries which feed the heart), cause a momentary drop in oxygen to the heart and an intense pain resembling that of angina pectoris (pseudo-anginal pain). The continual pains and the thoracic oppression appear to be linked to the constriction of the skeletal muscles, the constant state of tension of which causes distress. The increase in adrenalin secretion which accounts for the tachycardia and the extra systoles felt by the patients, is similarly a cause for pain and anxiety.

All these symptoms frequently bring spasmophilics to the cardiologist. However the cardiovascular examination is normal, and so too is the electrocardiogram (electrical tracing of the heart). The cardiologist is then able to say, in all good faith, that the consultant has a healthy heart and no cardiovascular disease. He will then mention pain linked to anxiety, "nervous" pain, but often without going further and without making a diagnosis of spasmophilia. The patient still has his pains and goes elsewhere in search of relief.

However, at times, in spite of the negative result of the basic cardiological examination (clinical examination and the electrocardiogram), the cardiologist might go further in his specialized exploration. He might have several reasons for doing this : either by virtue of proper professional concern not to overlook a specific lesion or in response to the insistence of a patient, who refuses to admit without explanation that his symptoms have no foundation, or because of a desire to affirm his authority over the patient, or possibly to "cover" himself against a highly improbable omission and confirm his status as consultant.

It is then that the spasmophilic commences a round of cardiological investigations, which are always costly to the patient and society, often distressing and painful, and sometimes dangerous, and hospitalization might even be required. Eventually surgical intervention is not ruled out and may be suggested to the spasmophilic as a possible remedy, though the absolute necessity for this has not been proved.

No one will deny the immense strides and interest in cardiovascular explorations, or the undeniable and beneficial success of surgery for cardiovascular lesions. Things must however be put in their proper perspective and the consultant should know the significance of spasmophilia in the etiology of chest pains, and how to make the diagnosis and treat spasmophilia in a patient in whom nothing else is found, before proceeding to acts of much greater consequence and compelling necessity.

# SPASMOPHILIA AND THE RESPIRATORY SYSTEM

Among the localizations of spasmophilic symptoms in the deep organs, the attack on the respiratory system is almost always present. These patients frequently describe such an attack as akin to a feeling of being caught in a vice. Breathing is often rapid, short and sometimes badly synchronized. These patients, instead of bringing into play the diaphragm which is the main muscle of the respiratory function, make particular use of the intercostal muscles and the neck muscles. This lack of synchronization accounts for the impression these patients give of panting. We also know that this rapid and superficial respiration is in itself a factor of alkalosis which maintains neuromuscular stimulation.

The sensations of pain and thoracic oppression are linked to spasms of the voluntary muscles and also to the smooth musculature (involuntary) of the bronchial. These bronchial spasms can produce whistling breathing which is extremely distressing and resembles asthma attacks (pseudo-asthmatic respiration). Apart from this, we are aware of the relationship that can exist between an authentic allergic asthma and spasmophilia.

The respiratory tree also includes the pharynx and the larynx. The localization of muscular spasms at this point is also entirely habitual. It is often even one of the symptoms that the patients describe to begin with : their "ball in the throat". This ball in the throat should not be mistaken for a symptom of anxiety, even if it is aggravated by anxiety. The ball in the throat is a constriction, a contraction of the pharyngeal muscles which can be painful and certainly alarming in itself. It is a symptom that can deeply trouble these patients, for the neck and the throat are parts of the body which are very sensitive and highly innervated.

Moreover, the impression of a tightening in the throat could suggest a goiter (chronic enlargement of the thyroid gland), creating even more panic for people who are already in a very anxious state.

The constriction of the pharyngeal muscles is accompanied by difficulty in swallowing, because a spasm of the upper part of the digestive tube (esophagus) is often associated with this. Here too, the fear of serious illness is extremely frequent. If the "ball in the throat" is a well known manifestation and physicians know more or less how to play it down, it is not always attributed to spasmophilia itself and all too often is considered to be a symptom of anxiety, whereas in many cases it is simply a secondary manifestation of anxiety.

The other respiratory manifestations of spasmophilia, however, frequently go unrecognized; they are nevertheless essential features to this illness, in particular because of the hyperventilation they engender.

The attack of the larynx which is the organ of the voice, enters into the framework of the respiratory localizations; the vocal chords which modulate sound are muscles. These muscles, like all the muscles of the human organism can be affected by neuromuscular stimulation, bringing about changes in the voice; the muffled voice, the broken voice, a permanent hoarseness, difficulty in the emission of certain sounds. Voice disturbances generally call for special tests, which if they are negative, should lead to spasmophilia being considered as a possible cause.

Finally, the dry mouth and frequent yawning must be added to the respiratory manifestations of the illness.

## SPASMOPHILIA AND THE DIGESTIVE SYSTEM

The digestive manifestations of spasmophilia are numerous and highly significant. Since the digestive tract has an obvious nutritional role, it has a causative role, as well which is no less important.

Spasmophilics are patients who don't eat or who overeat, who are constipated or who have diarrhea, who vomit or who suffer from the abdomen. The abdominal pains are very varied, ranging from permanent discomfort and dull pain to acute colic. They have chronic functional attacks of the colon. These disturbances of the alimentary canal bring on obesity or underweight. The diarrhea can cause actual dehydration. Constipation brings on pain and distaste for food. Gastric pains, regurgitation, abdominal distension, aerophagie and difficulties in swallowing caused by dyskinesia of the esophagus, are likewise very frequent.

Hepatic pain - pain of the bile ducts caused by spasms of the bilio-duodenal sphincter (the Oddi sphincter) or by the atony or hypertony of the gallbladder, completes this symptomatology.

In the course of a thorough investigation in search for a macrolesional organic illness all these digestive manifestations will result in common negative findings. This contrasts with the fact that there are clear-cut spasmophilia symptoms. These patients represent at least half of those who consult specialists in digestive pathology.

Symptoms concerning the colon are certainly the most numerous. It is well known that this organ is in a state of constant reactivity and has been compared to an "abdominal brain".

The wall of the colon is highly innervated with an autonomous nervous system and it is a choice area for the digestive manifestations of spasmophilia. These manifestations lead to many and useless therapies, repeated additional investigations and often a difficult relationship between the patient and his physician.

In this case, however, an X-ray of the colon, using a product for contrast (barium enema) shows specific aspects. Indeed, while showing the absence of any macroscopic organic lesion, the barium enema shows up the hyper-reactivity of the organ and the muscular spasms that contract it. The colon seems to appear as a "pile of dishes". The gastro-enterologists are familiar with these colic manifestations of neuromuscular stimulation. Many terms such as "spasmodic colitis", "neurogenic mucous colitis", "unstable colon", "irritable colon", "vulnerable colon", "spastic colon", "psychosomatic colopathie", have been made use of to name this condition.

But although the functional pathology of the colon has been known and recognized for a long time, few practitioners are concerned by the real microlesional mechanism that maintains it. In this mechanism, spasmophilia plays an important role by way of neuromuscular hyperexcitability and the hypersecretion of adrenalin. To diagnose a "functional colopathie" is one thing, to reassure the patient is of course necessary, and to eliminate a cancer is mandatory. But the diagnostic and therapeutic procedure should go further. And the recognition and treating of the spasmophilia, so often the causal agent of these troubles, is truly going further.

What is customarily referred to as the "hepatic terrain" is likewise part of the problems one generally comes up against in gastroenterology. The digestive manifestations of spasmophilia are in large part responsible. The relation between the liver and behavior dates back to antiquity. Symbolically speaking, "to be bilious", "to pour out one's bile", etc. are some of the expressions. Melancholia means black bile, that is to say, toxic. The first cause that comes to mind of people concerning jaundice is fear or emotion. Nevertheless this "hepatic terrain", recognized from childhood on in the patient, including distressing digestion, vomiting, migraine, pain in the right hypochondrium, has a very vague definition biologically, because the mechanisms of the hepatic function are difficult to penetrate by the most varied biological examinations. Only the specific symptoms of spasmophilia are very often present.

In the framework of manifestations termed "hepatic", the symptoms concerning the gall bladder and the bile ducts are the most frequent. The bile duct, outside of any gallstone pathology {gall bladder stones) may not contract sufficiently. The bile duct (which evacuates the bile from the gall bladder to the intestine) is likewise subject to variations in diameter; similarly and more especially, the Oddi sphincter (the circular muscle at the extremity of the bile duct). All these structures are extremely sensitive to a hypertonic spasm which causes pain and bile retention. The dependence on emotion of these bile dyskinesias (disturbance in the motor functioning) by the mechanism of neuromuscular stimulation in spasmophilia, is equally obvious.

The problem of food behavior (anorexia and bulimia) certainly concerns the digestive system, but it would seem preferable to discuss this under the heading of psychic manifestations of spasmophilia.

## SPASMOPHILIA AND RHEUMATOLOGY

Neuromuscular hyperstimulation manifests itself at the skeletal muscles in the form of spasms and rigid contractions. These spasms and rigid contractions are the source of various pains which often bring spasmophilics to consult with rheumatologists.

This concerns muscular pain which can be intense and can be seated all along the spinal column or at the level of the limbs.

In the neck the contractions of the nape of the neck cause pain and sensations of weight. There are also headaches that are seated at the rear of the cranium which may be either dull or stabbing. The pain can radiate all over the head and even to above the eyes.

In the back the pain is located between the shoulder blades and makes work in a sitting position extremely uncomfortable; it is described as a piercing pain accompanied by a deep lassitude.

In the lumbar region the pain can be dull or violent reaching an acute lumbago which forces the patient to stay in bed; it is made worse by effort and can make walking difficult. It can be complicated by painful radiations to the lower limbs resulting in unilateral or bilateral sciatica.

In the upper limbs the pain is diffused, accompanied by cramps, muscular fatigue, and difficulty in carrying heavy objects.

The pain can be intense and isolated, at the level of the lower limbs, accompanied by pain in the calves, sensations of compression of the feet, tingling in the toes.

In all the cases, the rheumatological tests are negative and the X-rays of the skeleton   are normal or show minor lesions, banal and static, with the rigid contraction alone being responsible for the pain and functional crippling. In contrast, the symptoms   associated   with   spasmophilia   are present, more especially fatigue.

The diagnosis of spasmophilia must not be lost sight of, for in all these cases analgesic and anti-inflammatory medication will have only a temporary effect. Similarly, manipulations of the vertebrae which do not displace them, but act only at the point of the localized contraction, will only help temporarily.

Rheumatologists and physicians who have specialized in functional re-education usually know that one must look for spasmophilia when confronted by pain of the spine and limbs which do not involve rheumatologic lesions. They know that their treatment will not have a lasting effect until such time as spasmophilia is diagnosed and properly treated as such and until the vicious circle pain-contraction has finally been broken.

Here again, spasmophilia must not be neglected or allowed to go unrecognized, because with persistent pain, particularly lumbar, there is a risk of additional traumatic complementary explorations, and a real dependence of the patient on certain physicians who practice vertebral manipulations, and who are always ready to give spectacular relief to some new contraction.

The pain in the spinal column has properly been called the "illness of the century" {one more !) and it is likely that it is one of the common forms of expression of spasmophilia.

Certainly rheumatological lesions do exist but, even in these cases, the contractions are often the main painful factor {we will see how spasmophilia aggravates the painful manifestations of arthritis), and spasmophilia is often found at the origin of these contractions.

The high social cost of arthritic pathology is well known and in this connection especially the treatment and prevention of spasmophilia is of significant interest.

## SPASMOPHILIC CHILDREN

For several reasons, it is necessary to deal specifically with spasmophilic children :

They are often "problem children" throughout their growth ; they are often children born into families of spasmophilics.

It is a propos of spasmophilic children that the problems of detection and prevention of spasmophilia present themselves most acutely.

This short chapter deals in particular with the spasmophilic child ; indeed, everything relating to the specific symptoms of the malady applies equally to children.

Spasmophilic children are often "problem children" who show disturbances in character; difficult children, intolerable or, as opposed to this, lifeless, apathetic, fatigued youngsters. They may have difficulties in adapting to school, which in turn has a repercussion on their schoolwork and their industriousness.

They can be irascible, aggressive and violent and often sleep too little or too much.

Children with difficult characters often have a childhood studded with pathological incidents.

In early infancy they may have had febrile convulsions {convulsions relating to a high fever) or sobbing spasms (fainting during a crying spell). These manifestations rightly worry their parents but tests, in particular electroencephalograms, are reassuring and eliminate the fear of epilepsy.

As they grow older they frequently have mild illnesses. They are the type of children who are often taken to a physician. Spasmophilic children have, it would appear, more accidents than others, doubtless because they are more nervous and inattentive.

With them, too, obesity and underweight are often observed, as well as constipation.

As for preadolescents and adolescents, spasmophilia manifests itself in the form of headaches and fatigue which can be linked to deterioration in schoolwork. As previously indicated, character difficulties are frequent and aggravate the problems that come at puberty.

Many spasmophilic children have brothers and sisters who also have the disease, and one just can imagine the daily life of these families of children, restless or apathetic, muddle-headed, fatigued and suffering from lack of sleep. The family character of spasmophilia is indisputable, and often one or both parents have the same illness which further amplifies the different problems that arise. Of course, these "nervous" or problem children are frequently taken to doctors and in such cases too, there is a great temptation to prescribe various sedatives or tranquilizers, because the exasperated parents usually demand them. However, it is necessary to recognize spasmophilic children and to treat them as such.

The prevention of spasmophilia is especially vital in the case of children, as their metabolic needs are greater during growth. Their needs are at least three times as great as the norm. These points will be developed in the chapter on the prevention of the illness.

## SPASMOPHILIA AND DERMATOLOGY

Dermatology is that branch of medicine which specializes in the study of skin diseases. The skin is one of the primary areas where the relationship between a macrolesional organic pathology and a microlesional functional pathology manifests itself and we will see that spasmophilia is bound up with many of the various disturbances of the cutaneous coating.

There are many reasons why spasmophilia has a predilection for affecting the skin:

1.      The skin plays a big part in the expression of emotions; one blushes with shame, becomes white with anger, and sweats with fear. The vasomotor and secreting phenomena that take place on the skin are components of the subject's emotions.

2.      The skin has a role of protective symbolism. This protective function is represented by the "frontier" with the outside world and is also most likely linked to the memory of the security conferred by the mother.

3.      The skin has an erogenous role that is well known.

4.      Lesions of the skin, because they are so blatant and have an unaesthetic character are particularly apt to have repercussions on the patient's psyche.

However, and this is a paradox, it is often the patients who have pathological cutaneous manifestations who are the most reticent or the most hostile to accepting the idea of there having been an emotional basis for the genesis of their troubles.

One of the most common symptoms is that of pruritus, namely, itching accompanied by the need to scratch oneself. These itches are often purely itches, without any objective cutaneous manifestation. They can affect the whole body in a varying way or may be localized at different areas of the body, at the external genital organs (vulvar pruritus) or at the anus. Spasmophilia is often detected in such patients who suffer from a pruritus (after having, of course, eliminated all other possible causes) and the treatment of the spasmophilia is usually successful.

Differing from pruritus, where there are no objective cutaneous manifestations, are other attacks on the skin accompanied by the presence of dermatological lesions. To begin with, this concerns, firstly, physiological manifestations such as a reddening which, if it becomes chronic, can develop into a real symptom such as acne rosacea (permanent distension of the blood vessels of the face).

Disturbances in the chronic functioning of the sweat-glands produce cold sweat, sometimes very profuse and really embarrassing; excessive perspiring of the hands, armpits, feet.

Other manifestations are more clearly pathological :

- Herpes   is a viral dermatosis in connection with which it has been known for some time that the recurrences are related to various emotions.

- Furunculosis, which is a microbial dermatosis, can resist all classical therapy, but is often associated with a depressive condition in relationship to a surge of spasmophilia.

- In juvenile acne, the role of sexual hormones and of overinfection is important, but certain typical manifestations of spasmophilia, such as fatigue and anxiety, are also frequently present, and here too, the treatment must very often be combined.

- Allergic dermatoses: eczema, urticaria are linked to specific allergies, but the sensitivity to the allergens varies considerably as a function of the emotional tension and spasmophilia is often present. The treatment of this spasmophilia most likely does not change the allergic terrain, but allows the subjects concerned to come into contact with harmful allergens without presenting pathological phenomena.

- Psoriasis is a recurrent cutaneous ailment usually a cause for despair for those who have it, sending them from one physician to another. A spasmophilia is often detected in these patients, and the treatment, if it does not cure the psoriasis, often helps to space out the recurrences and to reduce them. The maladies of the scalp (seborrhea, baldness, loss of hair) outside of their particular components, engender surges where the role of the emotions, emotional shocks, overwork, is clear-cut. Here too, a spasmophilia is often recognizable and should be treated as such.

All these facts militate in favor of looking for a spasmophilia in the face of various types of dermatological manifestations.

The treatment of the spasmophilia, if it is present, is the only mean for lasting cures, in conjunction with proper dermatological therapies.

# SPASMOPHILIA, STOMATOLOGY
# AND OTO-RHINO-LARYNGOLOGY

The mouth, nose, throat and ears can be the seat of numerous symptoms which, although they have no precise local cause, are frequently connected with spasmophilia.

In the mouth, glossodynias are localized pains often intense, without symptoms of irritation or lesion of the tongue or the teeth.

Dry mouth, and the contrary, hyper-salivation frequently occur in relation to sympathetic disturbances.

Bruxism (grinding of the teeth) is often encountered in spasmophilics and can cause lesions of the tooth enamel which are sometimes difficult to treat. This bruxism is something which can be exasperating for the family and friends of the spasmophilic.

The symptoms that concern the ears are disturbances of the equilibrium and hearing.

The attack on the equilibrium which borders on neurological pathology, manifests itself in spasmophilics by sensations of vertigo, instability in walking, the impression of walking in a fog. Aggravation of the disturbance provokes a more or less permanent fear of falling down, of an accident. This condition maintains the anxiety of patients and increases it to the point where some of them suffer from a state of depression. The cause of this is the labyrinthic hyper-reflectivity of the spasmophilic.

In the absence of any trace of neurological lesion, true rotating vertigos (vertigo of Meniere) also exist. These attacks of vertigo may force the patient to remain in bed, as he is unable to stand up without falling down. Everything around him turns, generally in the same direction. The spasmophilic terrain of these patients is always clear-cut with a pronounced anxiety, a past history of migraines and digestive disturbances. The vertigo attack is triggered by emotional stress or an occasional complication in daily life.

Tinnitus is a buzzing noise in the ears, whistling, or snoring, which can affect one or both ears. Very often no neurological or circulatory cause is detected as the origin for these tinnitus and they are regarded as relating to a neuralgic manifestation of the cochlea brought on by neuromuscular hyperstimulation.

The rhino-pharyngeal manifestations (of the throat and the nose) of spasmophilia can be part of the warning symptoms of the illness, since this is a sensorial zone par excellence with a rich neurovegetative innervation.

Spasmophilics complain of difficulty in swallowing their saliva, however during meals this does not happen and the pharyngeal discomfort disappears. They also complain of abnormal sensations, of a foreign body the localization of which varies from time to time. Sometimes they feel a disturbance of the nasal permeability. Certain spasmophilics complain of a permanent post-nasal drip coming from the back of the nose and dropping into the throat.

Finally, patients often describe the well known "ball in the throat", which is a constriction of the pharyngeal muscles, when they talk of their anxieties.

Likewise, a tingling in the throat (pharyngeal paresthesias) is often encountered.

In all these cases anxiety and hyper-emotivity are prominent and considerably aggravate these manifestations. The accompanying ear nose and throat examination is negative, or at the most, shows only slight lesions; a chronic tonsillitis, a minimal sinusitis, sometimes occasional allergic reactions.

The local treatment of these minor complaints does not suffice to cure the patient and the spasmophilia has to be treated, while patiently explaining the origin of these disturbances.

## SPASMOPHILIA AND OPHTHALMOLOGY

The neuromuscular excitability and the metabolic disturbance of spasmophilia have precise repercussions on the eyes and on the vision.

In the case of the eyes there are trophic disturbances of the crystalline lens which can cause an actual cataract. This cataract shows itself by fuzzy images, then by a reduction in visual acuteness which can develop into real blindness, calling for the surgical ablation of the disturbed crystalline lens.

Ophthalmologists are usually aware of these endocrine cataracts which answer to precise criteria. It refers to a cataract in the posterior capsule where the lesions commence at the posterior face of the crystalline lens due to a deposit of calcium. There are other causes besides spasmophilia for endocrine cataracts but spasmophilia is one of the principle etiologies and the rule is to request an electromyogram for such a lesion, particularly if it concerns a young person.

Cataracts generally appear at a relatively advanced age and are unusual between the ages of 20 and 40. If the spasmophilia is not recognized or not treated, the cataract develops unrelentingly until blindness, and becomes bilateral.

Likewise, if the treatment is undertaken too tardily, a surgical cure is often the only one possible. The cataracts of spasmophilia appear quite often in young women during their pregnancy or following it, which makes it imperative to correct the metabolic disturbances linked to the pregnancy. The treatment of the spasmophilia prevents the appearance of the crystalline lens disturbances or halts their development.

Other disturbances of the vision are linked to spasmophilia but less often recognized, because they are connected with a less serious pathology. They manifest themselves by way of fuzzy images caused by a disturbance of the convergence of the eyes and having their origin in spasms of the small muscles which ensure the movement of the eyes. Also through sensations of flies or bright spots in front of the eyes, difficulty in fixing objects, and episodes in which the subjects see double images (diplopia).

In certain strabismus (eyes that squint) spasmophilia likewise plays a role in the lack of coordination of the motor muscles of the eyes.

Transitory amaurosis constitutes rather frequent symptoms. These are episodes of sudden loss of vision in one or both eyes and which can last from a few seconds to several hours. These problems are particularly upsetting for the patients and ophthalmologists give them the greatest attention. Patients are often hospitalized for risky investigational procedures (arteriograms) to see if there is any obstacle to the circulation of arterial or venous blood. Now that many eye specialists are aware that spasmophilia can be responsible for these amaurosis, they often content themselves with simpler and less traumatizing conjunctive investigations, in particular, the Doppler velocimetry (study of the cerebral circulation by means of ultrasound) to eliminate the possibility of vascular lesion.

Finally, eyelids that blink or jump (palpebral clonias) continually or in occasional attacks, are frequent among spasmophilics and motivate them to consult with an ophthalmologist.

## SPASMOPHILIA AND GYNECOLOGY

Spasmophilia was first described and studied in women. We have dealt with this predominance, but it still remains true that the manifestations of neuromuscular hyperstimulation in gynecology are extremely numerous.

There is no intention to restrict ourselves to the psychological aspect of "women's diseases", but to understand that most reasons for consulting a gynecologist have a pathological basis. Here again this pathology is termed "functional", and involves to a large extent the specific mechanisms of spasmophilia.

The great frequency of problems of functional pathology, microlesional in women and more especially in the gynecological domain, is due to numerous physiological, pathological or emotional aggressions, specific in women which subsist throughout their lives.

Physiological aggressions are a natural part of women's lives:

- beginning of the menstruation and the morphological modifications of puberty ;

- normal modifications of the menstrual cycle under the neurohormonal dependence ;

- pregnancy and confinement, possibly breast-feeding, which are physically trying and bring about metabolic and hormonal upheavals in the organism ;

- spontaneous or voluntary abortions which, even excluding the more or less distressing nature of the experiences, are equally a source of hormonal storms ;

- menopause, finally, which can be felt as the beginning of ageing and can be a source of psychopathological accidents.

The pathological aggressions are likewise more numerous in women than in men :
   - disturbances of hormonal balance ;
   - cysts, fibromas and endometrioses ;
   - tumoral processes of the uterus, ovaries and breasts ;
   - genital infections after confinement or abortion.

The psycho-emotional aggressions too, have an impact : the effect of fear, emotion, moral suffering at the appearance or stopping of menstruation or on the production of leukorrheas (white secretions) and painful states.

Gynecologists estimate that of the women who consult them, a little more than 30% evidence macroscopic organic disturbances (fibromas, cysts, cancers, prolapse, etc.) and the remaining 70% have no visible macrolesion. A simple enumeration of the symptoms in which for the most part spasmophilia appears as a cause, gives an understanding of the dimensions of the problem :

- the disturbances of menstruation are the most typical - amenorrhea (absence of the menses) or dysmenorrhea (painful menses) ;

- pelvic pain, pain in the perineum, anorectal neuralgias ;

- pruritus (itching) of the vulva and cystalgias (pain during urination) without urinary infection ;

- the leukorrheas (the whites) without any infectious factor ;

- dyspareunia (painful contraction of the vagina) and frigidity, which will be discussed later;

- "inflammation" of the ovaries, a vague term, which, in fact, masks polycystic ovarian dystrophya which manifests itself by pain in the lower abdomen or the kidneys, irregularity of the menstrual cycle, a painful ovulation. The examination shows enlarged ovaries, heavy and painful, and it is known that this dystrophy is linked to psycho-emotional worries and family or social conflicts.

Pregnancy is often complicated and distressing in spasmophilic women with an incomplete loss of consciousness : malaises which are either lipothymias or syncope or spasmodic vomiting. After confinement, these women remain very fatigued for several weeks. Trophic troubles of the fingernails, teeth and hair manifest themselves, and also sometimes during pregnancy or after confinement, there are changes in the crystalline lens (see above).

It can be easily understood that during pregnancy, and afterwards, during breast feeding, if it is practiced, the ionic needs of the organism increase considerably and the spasmophilia must be recognized and treated during these periods.

Although most of the feminine sterilities have visible organic causes (obstruction of the tubes, insufficient ovarian secretions, anomalies of the uterine wall) a certain number, however, can only be explained by a hyper-motricity of the tubes or the uterus, which shortens the stay of the egg which cannot then be impregnated.

Likewise many repeated spontaneous abortions of healthy young women without uterine lesions, are without doubt, due to spasms of the uterine muscle which expels the fetus too soon.

In all these cases, the gynecological symptoms of neuromuscular hyperexcitability are associated with general symptoms which are important to find. It is only in this way that a great part of what is called "functional gynecological pathology" can be treated at a stage where the microlesions are not serious and are still reversible.

## THE SEXUAL LIFE OF SPASMOPHILICS

The sexual life of spasmophilics is often dramatic, punctuated by failures and despair. These patients certainly constitute the major proportion of the clients of sexologists, as much for the problems of the couple as for the sexual problems more peculiar to the man or the woman.

The repercussion on the genital sphere of the neuromuscular hyperexcitability and the anxiety it engenders and maintains, explains a good number of symptoms met with in sexual pathology ; firstly, the problems of the couple (for often spasmophilias marry each other, doubtless because they have similar psychological structures and as the saying goes, "birds of a feather flock together").

If life is already painful for a spasmophilic, fatigued, anxious, losing sleep, irritable, a prey to malaises, one can imagine what the daily life of a spasmophilic couple can be like, each one observing the other and the condition of one influencing the condition of the other.

Moreover, the surges of decompensation of the spasmophilia do not necessarily occur at the same time for both partners and one can feel well when the other is ill, which can cause rancor and resentment. One spasmophilic in a couple is often difficult to endure and the spouses of spasmophilics are well aware of this, but the life of a spasmophilic couple can be close to purgatory.

The problem of relations of the couple, already numerous, are aggravated by the sexual difficulties peculiar to spasmophilics.

In women, dyspareunia (contraction of the vaginal muscles) and frigidity are very frequent.

Dyspareunia is a permanent contraction of the constrictor muscles of the vagina which makes penetration painful, and even impossible. Muscular spasms and anxiety are directly responsible for this rigid contraction. Dyspareunia can cause women to refuse sexual relations or to space them out through fear of pain and because these relations are rarely satisfactory. The sexual act may be shortened, considered as a chore or even felt as rape. This is not a matter of mental attitude, but truly a physical suffering, making an act, which is supposed to give pleasure, unbearable.

Frigidity is the impossibility of obtaining an orgasm : it may be accompanied by an absence of sexual desire. Here again, this may be caused by muscular spasms, the impossibility of relaxing, the pain and anxiety as well as the lack of being in the mood for sex. The partner of a spasmophilic woman does not remain indifferent, and his reactions can go from resentment to exasperation, and eventual lack of interest.

All these reasons explain why spasmophilic women are rarely satisfied sexually, even with suitable partners. The lack of sexual satisfaction is in itself a source of anxiety and increases the instability and depressive nature of these patients.

The most frequent disturbances with male spasmophilics are premature ejaculation and impotence.

Premature ejaculation is characterized by normal erection which does not last, and the masculine orgasm, that is the ejaculation of the sperm, arriving rapidly or in any case, too rapidly for the woman to find for herself the rhythm of the sexual act and reach orgasm. The ejaculation occurs rapidly at the slightest solicitation, sometimes even before penetration, during the preliminary contacts. This premature ejaculation cannot be controlled and is linked to the neuromuscular hyperexcitability. In addition, the anxiety of the premature ejaculation, not satisfying the partner, and not being a valid partner, aggravates matters further and makes the control of the erection more difficult.

Impotence is the absence of erection or an insufficient erection to allow penetration. The fatigue of spasmophilics rarely seems to be in question and it is likely that the impotence has a central mechanism, linked to anxiety. The fear of being unable to have an erection prevents the erection from occurring. The depression of the spasmophilic, likewise, intervenes with a loss of interest in sexual relations.

Impotence is always accepted with difficulty by spasmophilics. They either resent their partner for not stimulating them sufficiently, or else they have reactions of shame. In any case, the subject feels impotence as a deep wound to the ego, and has grievous consequences on the relationship of the couple.

An example of the problems of impotence for spasmophilics is as follows :

Mr. J., a 48 years old decorator, had a normal sexual life until his wife left him. After this separation a state of permanent fatigue set in, to which were added preoccupying problems (including a petition for bankruptcy of his firm). But overall, while retaining the desire for sexual relations, he had become impotent. This condition varied somewhat with different partners but was usually almost total. Mr. J. felt guilty and even entertained thoughts of suicide. However his organic sexual function was intact since he often awoke in the morning with an erection. He had consulted several sexologists and had undertaken several treatments, one of which was a psychoanalytically oriented psychotherapy lasting for several years without appreciable results.

The association of a depressive condition, asthenia, sexual difficulties, and the presence of clear-cut triggering factors then brought to mind the possibility of spasmophilia. Additional examinations confirmed this diagnosis and after 4 months of treatment, Mr. J. progressively recovered a satisfactory sexual functioning which he has now maintained for four years.

Premature ejaculation and impotence for men with spasmophilia often makes them very poor sexual partners.

Dyspareunia and frigidity in women with spasmophilia often make them unbearable sexual partners.

The various possible combinations of spasmophilic couples are easy to imagine and many anecdotes could be told. In all these cases, spasmophilia causes drama, sexual dissension, and the life of the couple or simply, the relationship is seriously disturbed.

# SPASMOPHILIA AND PSYCHE

The psychic manifestations of spasmophilia are without doubt the least understood, and this often brings about unwarranted psychiatric treatment, and the ignoring of related problems which are easily cured.

However, before discussing the psychic manifestations proper to the disease, it is well to point out that there exists a true neurological symptomatology. The neurological symptoms of spasmophilia are associated in various degrees ; fainting which may be preceded by malaise, instability when walking and sensations of dizziness, impressions of having an empty head, disturbances in states of consciousness, disturbances in vision, clumsiness and trembling of the extremities, and finally attacks of tetany.

This indeed involves a neurological pathology, that is, one that concerns the central and peripheral nervous system in its functioning, its efficacy and its performance, without bringing in the matter of psychological functions.

In all these cases the classical complete neurological examination is normal except for the symptoms proper to neuromuscular overstimulation and neurologists cannot point to a precise syndrome in relation to one or several structures of the nervous system. Here too, the highly elaborate methods of diagnostic neurological investigations can show no organic macrolesion. The loss of consciousness is often preceded by malaise, haziness in front of the eyes, difficulty in breathing, tingling in the mouth and the extremities, numbness.

The patient then faints, that is, falls down unconscious. The total loss of consciousness can last a few seconds to several minutes. During this loss of consciousness the patient is usually relaxed, limp, hypotonic. He can hurt himself when falling, but there is almost never biting of the tongue or loss of urine.

Although the existence of early symptoms is an excellent sign of spasmophilia, there can also be a real loss of consciousness without any premonitory symptom and which can last several tens of minutes.

In these latter, cases of macro-organic neurological lesions will be investigated immediately and therefore where spasmophilics are concerned, the findings will be negative.

Instability in walking is described as the sensation of being drunk, to lurch in walking, sometimes seeing objects turning. This instability which can be very embarrassing, often causes falls and can limit the activity of the patient.

The impressions of empty-headedness may be accompanied by loss of memory, difficulty in finding words, difficulties in articulation and also disturbances in the states of consciousness, in particular, drowsiness and problems of concentration.

We have seen that problems in vision include impressions of hazy images, difficulties in fixing objects, and impressions that the lines and words jump when reading.

The trembling of the extremities can be constant or aggravated by emotions and accompanied also by a sensation of internal trembling and jerking of the muscles. This trembling never has the character of symptomatic neurological trembling. Attacks of tetany have already been mentioned : these are strong attacks of intense and painful contractions of the limbs and the torso, altogether characteristic, which deform the hands into the "grip of the midwife" and stiffen the body into an arc of a circle.

All these neurological manifestations of neuromuscular overstimulation cause anxiety because they are impressive and very embarrassing and no reassuring explanation can be found for the patients.

They are therefore bound up with psychic manifestations proper to spasmophilia.

The psychic manifestations of the disease are most prominently characterized by anxiety and anguish. We have seen that this anxiety is a symptom of spasmophilia caused by various metabolic and humoral disturbances which exist in this disease and which act directly on the brain centers that control the emotions. It is only secondarily that the other symptoms of neuromuscular overstimulation cause anxiety by themselves and increase this pre-existing stress.

Spasmophilics are patients whose illness makes them anxious and whose anxiety, secondarily, aggravates the illness.

Anxiety is a constituent of spasmophilia and it can be defined as a painful affective condition which consists of a distressing expectation of a vague but imminent danger. This "fear without apparent cause" is accompanied by the physical symptoms of spasmophilia which are in reality the object and the real reasons of the fear. The anxiety is above all the result of feelings experienced ; the anguish, to a greater degree, is more the result of physical sensations.

Anguish is therefore created by somatic symptoms, oppression, and thoracic constriction, lack of air, tightening of the throat, rapid and irregular respiration, trembling, visual blurring, and the start can occur suddenly as an attack of anguish with an intense and uncertain fear, expectation of a vague catastrophe, a feeling of imminent death; the face is pale and covered with sweat, the features are drawn, the patient is either "paralyzed" by fear or agitated and feverish with tears and crying.

Chronic anxiety reproduces the same symptoms but less violently. The continual tension brings a feeling of insecurity. The simplest of matters is felt as threatening. The least malaise is seen as the symptom of a serious disease. The patient cannot take the slightest decision, and is in a constant state of doubt with feelings of failure and incapacity. The mood is unstable and the reactions to outside stimulations can be very sharp.

Here also the physical manifestations of excessive neuromuscular stimulation at the cardio-respiratory, digestive and neurological levels, are always present.

These chronic states of anxiety are often complicated by real depressive states with loss of the zest for life and mood disturbances: sadness, pessimism, feelings of inferiority, self-deprecation, even guilt.

The loss of the vital impulse takes the form of an overall slackening of pace, psychological and motor, which includes, particularly, a general fatigue, a total and progressive disinterest, loss of initiative, loss of intellectual efficiency and a reduction of motor activity. A feeling of total pessimism with tormenting ideas of inferiority, auto-depreciation and morbid sadness shows the depressive mood.

Disturbance of sleep is extraordinarily frequent in spasmophilia. There is more than one cause and several factors determine its appearance. Insomnia is one of the manifestations of anxiety states and depressive states. Muscular tension and pain disturb their sleep. An excessive production of adrenalin has a direct effect on the centers which regulate sleep.

We see then that there are many reasons why these patients sleep poorly. However, the insomnia of spasmophilics has very particular characteristics : the insomnia occurs in the second part of the night. The tired out patients fall asleep rapidly and sometimes even too rapidly. However, at about two or three in the morning, they wake after three or four hours of sleep and cannot fall asleep again. They are restless, toss in their bed and often have frightful nightmares with dreams of falling. This sort of insomnia of the second part of the night is quite different from the mental rumination which prevents the dropping off to sleep in patients who have anxious or depressive states in the psychiatric sense. This is an additional argument indicating spasmophilia, in which the psychic disturbances are secondary to metabolic disorders.

The psychic manifestations of neuromuscular overstimulation : anxiety, depressions and insomnia, often bring spasmophilics to consult psychiatrists and this is the start of many problems.

The great majority of specialists in mental illnesses do not recognize the existence of spasmophilia. For them, anxiety is a neurosis and the insomnias, neurotic symptoms. All the physical symptoms of spasmophilia are likewise laid at the door of mental disturbances. This attitude, if pushed to its limits, sees spasmophilia as a modern cultural form of hysterical neurosis.

The refusal to acknowledge a metabolic pathology, easily identifiable and curable, leads to many patients having to undergo psychiatric treatment. Such treatment ranges from the administration of chemotherapies, light or heavy, to unwarranted hospitalization in clinics or psychiatric hospitals, not forgetting various forms of psychotherapy involving varying degrees of analysis. Reinforced by the attitude of the psychiatrists, the close associates of these patients are only too ready to believe in mental illness and imaginary troubles.

To be considered mad is one more torment which afflicts spasmophilics for they are treated as mental cases by psychiatrists, and considered hypochondriacs by those near to them.

We have stopped counting the cases of spasmophilics who have languished for years in psychiatric hospitals and homes for mental patients, stunned by drugs, in despair but still lucid enough to understand their condition, before their metabolic disturbances were recognized and treated as such.

## STRESS AND SPASMOPHILIA

If "stress" is widespread in modern societies, and spasmophilia is likewise extremely frequent, is it feasible to assimilate these two notions ? In other words, are stress and spasmophilia "normal" forms of reaction of the organism reflecting poor adaptation to modern forms of civilization ?

This question is acute because it entails making of spasmophilia a clinical form for a normal person, the spasmophilic manner of facing the world. Certain physicians want to minimize or deny that it constitutes a metabolic disease.

The concept of stress has been studied by the Anglo-Saxon School, based on the work of Professor Hans Selye who is truly the father of this notion that he defines as a "non specific reply of the organism to any demand made upon it."

An emotion, in a wide sense, good or bad, produces in the organism a similar biological and hormonal response which is responsible for modifications which ensure adaptation at the level of various organs. This response of the organism can be good and adapted to the situation, or on the contrary, excessive and outstripping the organism's capacity for adaptation. The stress and the adaptation response to very dissimilar demands are termed "stress factors". The whole of the biological somatic, organic, functional and psychological manifestations provoked by an excessive response and exceeding the adaptation capacity of the organism, is called "stress condition". This stress condition is felt as a state of fatigue and exhaustion, lassitude and nervous tension.

We see here symptoms close to those described in spasmophilia, all the more so because the description of "stressed" persons allows us to recognize numerous symptoms with which we are familiar:

- A fatigue that occurs in the morning.

- Intellectual fatigue, memory lapses, a reduction in intellectual efficiency.
- Sexual fatigue, with a reduction of desire and difficulties in having an erection.
-   Stiffness and diffuse pain.
- Impatience, irritability, nervousness, anxiety, anguishes.
- Disturbances in social and family relationships.
- Headaches, migraine, palpitations, chest pains.
- Cramps and heartburn, diarrhea or constipation, loss of appetite or bulimia.
- Skin eruptions, itching, attacks of psoriasis or eczema.
- Disturbance in sleeping, frequently with early waking in the second part of the night.

It is therefore interesting and necessary to consider the relations that can exist between stress and spasmophilia, on the theoretical level as well as on the practical and therapeutic levels.

Before going into the possible connections between these two problems, it is necessary to describe briefly the present conceptions of stress. The state of chronic stress is today considered to be a disease of adaptation. The response of the organism to stress, that is, its adaptation to an aggression (or an emotion in a wide sense) is carried out by means of the nervous and endocrine systems.

The nervous system is represented here by the sympathetic system (vegetative nervous system) which is not under the control of the will and innervates the various organs (stomach, intestine, heart...) as well as the adrenal medulla gland. The sympathetic nervous system secretes adrenalin from the nerve fiber terminals and also from the medullary portion of the adrenal glands.

The endocrine system is especially represented here by the cortical portion of the adrenal glands which secrete cortisone. Adrenalin and cortisone are called stress hormones or adaptation hormones. As soon as some agent acts on the organism, a "message of stress" is set up which goes from the threatened region to the brain.

The response of the organism is carried out by the hypothalamo-hypophyseal path which is dependent on the limbic system. Two types of response to stress are known: an immediate response which is characterized by a secretion of adrenalin ; and a more tardy response, slower and continual, which comes from the secretion of cortisone.

The adrenalin frees the reserve of sugar which is stored in the liver - the sugar is necessary for the muscles and the brain. Adrenalin accelerates the heart rhythm, raises the arterial pressure and increases the circulation in the muscles and the brain. we have seen that the adrenalin likewise increases the excessive neuro-muscular stimulation.

The cortisone provokes the production of sugar in the liver by the breakdown of proteins, thus providing an easily available source of energy. It also reduces inflammation reactions.

One can then understand that in situations of chronic stress the adaptation and defense mechanisms end up by functioning in an abnormal manner, thus creating a whole pathological symptomatology.

After this brief outline of the Anglo-Saxon conceptions of stress, we can appreciate better the similarities and differences of stress and spasmophilia.

The similarities :

- the great resemblance of many symptoms, more especially those linked to muscular exhaustion and anxiety;
- the important role of adrenalin which is known for neuromuscular stimulation;
- it is also noteworthy that stress causes a leakage and an inactivation of magnesium due to the hormones of stress which liberate fatty acids, which in turn disactivate the magnesium. Those who work on stress describe the protective role of magnesium on the heart and the blood vessels, and the pathological consequences on the cardiac muscle by a deficit of magnesium. He will come back to this matter when discussing diseases that are aggravated by spasmophilia.

The differences :

- Stress, a disease of adaptation concerns all individuals having accumulated a certain number of "stress factors"; we know of course that although everyone undergoes stress, not everyone is spasmophilic.

- Authors treating stress insist on this accumulation from which it follows that the symptoms they describe strike especially at middle age, toward the forties. We know, however that spasmophilia exists at all age levels.

- A certain number of serious diseases linked to stress (ulcers of the stomach or the duodenum, myocardial infarction) are not part of the symptomatology of spasmophilia.

- Cortisone, whose role is important in the stress theory, is not in the forefront of the mechanisms of spasmophilia.

Summing up, if all the organisms respond in the same manner to stress factors, and can develop diseases of adaptation after an accumulation of stress factors, spasmophilia is a pathological entity that, although close, is different. The similarities are linked to certain common physiopathological mechanisms. The differences are linked to a notion of terrain, where the specificity of spasmophilia intervenes, the terrain for spasmophilia being doubtless linked, as we have seen, to a congenital disturbance of the permeability of the cellular membrane.

But it can certainly be said that spasmophilia, due to their constitutional fragility, are particularly exposed to stress. The mechanisms that produce the symptoms for stress and spasmophilia are close, so that their reactions will be stronger and more violent, and if the stress decompensates the spasmophilia, it is certain that spasmophilics are much more exposed to stress than non-spasmophilics. These considerations are important when we deal with the life hygiene of spasmophilics.

## DISEASES AGGRAVATED BY SPASMOPHILIA

The diseases aggravated by spasmophilia constitute a chapter the outline of which is necessarily schematic, and serves mainly to set down ideas for a layman. It isn't possible to give a true nosological classification, in this context.

On the one hand certain effects which are very diverse and poorly known can be discerned. These effects have in common a "functional" character, with neuromuscular overstimulation most probably playing a role. On the other hand there are well-defined autonomous effects where the existence of an associated spasmophilia plays an aggravating role.

The "functional" diseases where spasmophilia plays a role are specially represented by:

- The allergic disorders : asthma, eczema, urticaria, hay fever, and spasmodic coryza. These allergic disorders are the result of the reaction of the organism to a specific allergen, that is, in the presence of these allergens (house dust, cat hairs, flower pollen, etc.) the organism will manufacture specific antibodies producing an allergic reaction which manifests itself by one of the various ailments mentioned above. Now we know that spasmophilia is often present in allergic subjects; it is not the only factor but it complicates the symptoms and must therefore be treated conjointly with a specific desensitization.

- Essential hypertension of the young subject : hypertension (permanent increase of blood pressure above normal levels) can have multiple causes and physicians specialized in these complaints, use a number of complementary approaches to find a cause for this hypertension which is curable. However, particularly for young people, when no cause can be found for this rise in tension, it is regarded as "essential hypertension".

In such cases there is often a spasmophilia and it is felt that the prolonged spasm of the blood vessels is responsible. The spasm in fact reduces the caliber of the vessels and the blood pressure must rise to maintain a sufficient flow of blood. In addition, we have seen that an exaggerated secretion of adrenalin by itself increases the arterial pressure.

- The cyclic edemas : this concerns patients whose legs and sometimes arms swell and then subside (accumulation of water in the tissues) without any circulatory or general cause to explain this. spasmophilia is often present and its treatment improves or cures these symptoms.

- The functional hypoglycemias : hypoglycemias, that is, a drop of the sugar level of the blood, either permanent or in attacks, can certainly have macrolesional organic causes that are well known to physicians, but often no precise cause can be found. Here too, a spasmophilia is often present resulting from mechanisms which are still unknown. The problem of functional hypoglycemia is all the more interesting, considering that it also causes states of fatigue and sudden drops in energy. In particular, these people may have peaks of hypoglycemia which are sometimes quite pronounced some hours after they have eaten. The patients then experience fatigue and somnolence, even malaises, which may resemble spasmophilia to the point of seeming identical. It follows, consequently, that a hypoglycemia must be looked for when a spasmophilia is detected, and a spasmophilia should be looked for when a functional hypoglycemia is discovered. These are two metabolic disturbances which can be intimately linked.

- The thyroid dysfunction is a disturbance in the functioning of the thyroid gland, either because of excess or insufficient secretion. Outside of some well-defined organic lesions there is often no explanation for this dysfunction. An excessive secretion causes a loss of weight, fatigue, acceleration of the cardiac rhythm, diarrhea, insomnia, etc: Insufficient functioning causes obesity, hypothermia, loss of hair, constipation, etc.

All these symptoms are common to those of spasmophilia and very often an associated spasmophilia is detected in these patients without knowing the exact link between these two types of diseases, but here also, neither one should be neglected in the treatment.

In well-defined autonomous ailments, spasmophilia intervenes as an aggravating factor :

The cardiovascular diseases are aggravated by spasmophilia ; indeed, in many of these effects the diagnosis of the disease is linked to the obstruction of the blood vessels by the deposit of fat. To these complete or partial obstructions, are added spasms that temporarily reduce the caliber of the vessels causing partial or complete reductions in the circulation of the blood.

It is easy to understand the role of spasmophilia which increases the production of vascular spasms; these spasms, occurring in pathological vessels, may cause serious accidents. It has been determined that magnesium plays a protective role in the vessel walls against atheroma (clogging of the arteries by deposits of fat) by inhibiting the creation of blood clots in the arteries and the veins. The magnesium deficit of spasmophilics exposes them more to atheroma and the formation of clots.

Osteoporosis is also aggravated by spasmophilia. Osteoporosis is part of the aging processes of the bone structure characterized by a reduction of the calcium level. Osteoporosis causes bone pains and makes the bones fragile, sometimes causing spontaneous fractures or the shrinkage of the vertebras. We have seen that spasmophilia draws on the calcium in the bones to maintain a constant level of calcium in the blood. Spasmophilia promotes osteoporosis and adds to it when it has already started.

Alcoholism causes extremely serious and varied metabolic disorders, but all these disorders are aggravated in spasmophilics; in particular, the magnesium deficit makes the nerve cells more fragile and therefore more open to attacks which come from the abuse of alcoholic beverages.

Epilepsy is a disease of the brain which is characterized by specific lesions and which causes the well-known convulsive attacks. There are specific treatments for epilepsy which usually arrest the attacks and give patients the possibility of leading a normal life albeit with minor difficulties.

Spasmophilia may be associated with epilepsy and aggravate it. Treatment of spasmophilia often allows a better control of epilepsy and a reduction of the dosage of the specific anticonvulsive medication.

Hysteria is one of the authentic psychiatric neurotic manifestations. It is characterized by nervous attacks, disturbances of emotional life, staginess, erotomania, nymphomania, etc.

We have seen that in 10 to 15 per cent of cases, the psychic manifestations of spasmophilia are symptomatic of an anxiety neurosis or an hysteria neurosis, but the presence of an associated spasmophilia aggravates the condition of these neurotics and the treatment should be composite.

These few examples of diseases associated with spasmophilia or diseases in which it plays an aggravating role, illustrate once more the essential role of this disease and the presence of neuromuscular overstimulation in numerous pathological processes. These associations make it more than ever necessary to train physicians to have an overall view of disease in all its components, organic and functional.

III

## WHY CERTAIN PHYSICIANS DENY OR NEGLECT
## THE ROLE OF SPASMOPHILIA ?

The attitudes in the medical profession toward spasmophilia are extremely divergent and it is interesting to consider the many reasons for this.

Certain of these reasons are common to the entire profession ; various specialists hold others. We will examine particularly the position of the neuropsychiatrists.

The first reason for these divergences has to do with the rules in medical teaching. Since the beginning of the century, it has been the practice to divide the disturbances observed in pathology into functional symptoms and organic symptoms. This practice, instituted at the outset of medical studies and maintained later by the framework in which the studies are structured, favors privileged organic symptoms, that is, those that correspond to an identifiable anatomical lesion. It underplays functional symptoms, that is, those that do not correspond to sufficiently evident and visible anatomical lesions.

This conception has held sway in French medicine, and also, doubtless, in the technological medicine of all the developed countries, permeating the entire medical training. In the hospital it is habitual to present a patient as a "functional" case, thus politely indicating that he is not really ill but a "psychic" case, perhaps even a shammer. This way of thinking shapes clinical semiology (study and description of disease symptoms) which the student learns to recognize when examining a patient. Each of the clinical symptoms corresponds with a precise organic lesion. This lesion shows itself on the X-ray or the surgeon can see it or palpate it, or if the patient is less fortunate, it will be found in the course of an autopsy.

The search for the symptom of a lesion is the major preoccupation of physicians and controls their actions, consciously or unconsciously. It is clear that the lesion to be detected must be sufficiently important, or large. Organic pathology is based on macrolesions. The organ must be deeply injured for it to show up.

The fundamentalists (biochemists, physiologists, biophysicists) know of course the neurosecreting or molecular modifications of the organs before they are deeply injured but these specialists are the poor relatives of medicine, and although the fundamental sciences are part of medical teaching, they are regarded as the first obstacles in the race for a diploma, rather than truly creative disciplines. Disciplines cut off from practical medical reality are quickly forgotten when "serious matters" come up.

The present medical trend apparently gives priority to the research for fundamental causes of disease at the immunological or cellular level, but these avenues of research have as yet had little effect on the practical and everyday attitude of the medical profession which is directed towards research and treatment of the "macrolesion". It should be noted that the multiplicity of technological equipment with which modern medicine has armed itself is almost entirely oriented in this way. The most modern techniques and those using them, whether it concerns MRI, ultrasound or scanners, not to mention the numerous X-ray devices for producing contrasts, serve above all else to discover or eliminate a macrolesion. The discovery of a lesion constitutes the satisfaction of the physician. Proposing a new technology that will show up more lesions or reveal them more clearly is the objective of the diagnostic imagining of specialists in this field. The organic lesion constitutes a solid ground on which the physician can work. It shows itself and physicians present it to each other and treat it. It can be operated on. For these reasons, modern techniques of complementary investigation, are more and more techniques of visualization. The discovery of the image of the lesion is the development which the progress of medical diagnosis has followed in regard to the symptom of the lesion, which was previously the object of any investigation.

The obsession with the organic, of which the modern form is the search for the image of the lesion, has obscured the fact that pathology without a visible macroscopic organic lesion is nevertheless organic.

But this concerns minimal lesions at the cellular or metabolic level whose visualization is difficult or impossible. The organic nature of this microlesional pathology which shows itself by pathology in the functioning of the organs (functional pathology) has not yet become widely accepted.

The cult that modern societies devote to images is without doubt related somehow to this lack of recognition of the microlesion. In this sense it is fortunate that the neuromuscular overstimulation of spasmophilia can be visualized on a screen in the form of doublets or multiplets !

———

The priority given to the "organic", that is to the serious lesion, by medical training and thereafter by the usual practice of medicine, is the principle reason for the rejection of spasmophilia as a pathological entity by many doctors. The discredit attached to spasmophilia gives the feeling that a functional disturbance is not valid and that a patient predisposed to functional troubles is not to be taken seriously.

Other reasons figure in the rejection of spasmophilia by part of the medical profession. In particular, the uncertainty that still exists as to its mechanisms, for although many of the elements of this mechanism are known, others are still uncertain or mere hypotheses. Here too the need for simple straightforward explanations is felt. The uncertainties of the therapies have worked equally against spasmophilia. First calcium was put forward, then considered dangerous and abandoned ; magnesium then took the center of the stage. Different forms of vitamin D were boosted and then rejected. The uncertainty of the treatment went hand in hand with the uncertainty of the results. Improperly applied or insufficient treatments were of course not effective. Therefore spasmophilia is not treated, and a disease that is not treated is not a disease, etc. Moreover, spasmophilia is not a fatal disease, it is too mild to be dangerous, therefore too mild to be taken seriously. It should be noted that all these practitioners know little of the hell which many spasmophilics have to endure.

The attitude of various medical specialists arises in great part from the same reasons, accentuated by the fact that above all else, the specialists are technicians who are interested in a given system and do not look at the patient as a whole, as would the general practitioners. The search for a given lesion in a system is the "raison d'être" of the specialist who is supposed to be more expert in all the details proper to one or another pathology. It is for this reason that the general practitioner calls on him or that the patients consult him directly. Since he knows a sector of pathology better, the treatments that he prescribes are supposed to be more effective.

The specialist will further have a tendency to perform many diagnostic investigations in his field of competence, for it is expected of him that he knows all in his domain. The search for the lesion or the diagnosis becomes even more thorough and more elaborate. The credibility of the specialist rests on his technical skill.

The sector of the human body which is within his scope is examined from every angle before the verdict of a lesional diagnosis is rendered, or on the contrary, the specialist concludes that the supposed patient does not have a disease.

Neurologists usually have a similar attitude for they favor the organism and the lesion. This is even more so, because the neurological school is deeply influenced by the work of Babinski, who was able to describe precisely an entire clinical symptomatology corresponding to extremely precise anatomical lesions in the structure of the nervous system. The neurological pathology corresponds to specific attacks verified anatomically in one or another part of the central or peripheral nervous system, and apart from these attacks, here also there is only the "functional".

The spasmophilics are examined and treated by general practitioners or specialists who favor the organic (which is only the macrolesional) and forget, do not know, or do not want to know, that the functional is first of all microlesional.

Such physicians regard functional pathology as "psychic" and quite naturally, the spasmophilic will find himself among the psychiatrists. Psychiatrists have similar attitudes to spasmophilia, as exist among other categories of doctors, but these attitudes are reversed.

By a sudden turn around, psychiatrists interest themselves in the psyche, forgetting the physiological, that is the organic microlesional bases of the psychic symptoms of spasmophilics. For most of them, there are no spasmophilics whose metabolical disturbances bring about functional disturbances or symptoms with psychic expression, but on the contrary, these are patients having neuroses or depressive states. This too, is the result of a medical attitude which refuses to see the human being as a whole. Functional pathology, that is in the case of spasmophilia - microlesional pathology linked to a cellular and metabolic substratum - will be seen by these psychiatrists, either as a hysterical or anxiety neurosis, or a neurotic depression.

The functional manifestations are often arranged under the term of "conversion", for they presuppose that the symptoms have been created by the psyche. During the heyday of classical psychiatry, Charcot had shown that certain states of paralysis in hysterical patients were entirely psychic. These hysterical paralyses have gone out of style and psychiatrists feel that the various functional manifestations of spasmophilia are only the modern form taken by hysteria, once described by Charcot.

There certainly exist psychoses which are a true mental pathology. (I will not go into the rather arbitrary distinction that exists between neuroses and psychoses). In the case of psychoses one must recognize the immediate interest of various chemotherapies which have transformed the prognosis of true "madness". But beyond this serious pathology, the neuroses are in fact more or less    accentuated disturbances of behavior where the functional pathology of spasmophilia plays a large part.

These patients are the victims of psychiatric therapy. The same remedies are applied to the "insane" and to spasmophilics with, in the latter cases, frequently catastrophic results. The patients who annoy the doctors by their symptoms are "tranquilized", and then doped to offset their inertia.

This attitude of the psychiatrists confronted with spasmophilia and functional pathology in general, joined to the enormous array of medication available to modern psychiatry, explains why so many patients are saturated with various drugs. The research and treatments of microlesional organic symptoms are neglected in favor of treatment of mood disturbances by drugs acting on the mood. To make a simple comparison, this is like treating the pain from a decayed tooth by prescribing an aspirin rather than treating the tooth itself.

The classical medical attitude draws a distinction between organic pathology which is accessible to a lesional diagnosis and to specific therapies, and the functional pathology which is neglected or treated as a psychiatric symptom. Of course, this distinction has not escaped recognition as being inappropriate in many cases. The medical profession has turned to psychology, psychosomatics, even psychoanalysis with prudence and reticence. But people practicing these techniques also forget physiology or are unaware of it. The microlesional pathology escapes them, their approach to the total person remains timid. They act in an abstraction which is either tinged with an unacknowledged and unrecognized pathologism, or still worse, a poorly understood "psychoanalysism". The symptoms, in the case of spasmophilia are not ideas that some shoddy words will do away with, but are demonstrable and curable facts. The temptations of psychoanalysis and psychologism stir up mere wind and can prosper only in a medical practice which shies away from the problems of the patient as a whole person.

## SPASMOPHILIA IS AN AUTHENTIC DISEASE

Although certain physicians deny its existence, spasmophilia is an authentic disease. This statement is based on a list of several facts which it is useful to go over again :

Spasmophilia is defined by precise clinical symptoms, constant and easily recognizable.

The circumstances that triggered the always-characteristic disturbances are related during the clinical examination of patients presenting these symptoms..

The clinical symptoms, and particularly the electrophysiological criteria of the disease are indisputable.

The existence of cellular, ionic, metabolic and neuro-endocrine microlesions which cause neuromuscular overstimulation is well established, and the mechanisms that produce the symptoms have been largely explained.

The source of production of the symptoms is organic ; if a spasmophilic has pain, his body is not expressing psychic suffering, but a truly physical pain.

Spasmophilics know they are ill, they distinguish the period when they were in good health from the time they fell ill, their behavior is normal and their judgment sound. Their talk is logical, they try to face up to their illness and they want to be cured.

Finally, and this will be the subject of another chapter, the specific treatments of spasmophilia are remarkably efficient in at least 80 per cent of cases, and restore a normal life to patients who were often in despair.

Spasmophilia is not, therefore, a psychosomatic disease in the sense usually understood by this term ; a disease in which psychological problems create physical symptoms and disturbances. It is, on the contrary, a somato-psychic illness with an organic origin where metabolical disturbances create secondary psychic symptoms.

The existence of vicious circles which maintain and perpetuate the spasmophilia represents a perfect illustration of the concept certain authors have apropos diseases which are called psychosomatic, a term which they suggest should be written in a circular manner.

# THE ROLE OF THE PHYSICIAN

Before one is able to recognize spasmophilia, one must know what it is. However, the medical profession as a whole, fails to recognize this disease. This attitude can be either voluntary or involuntary. Involuntary at times because of lack of education and information, or insufficient education in dealing with the question. Also at times, because it concerns a pathology regarded as "minor", it is neglected by the classical medical education which applies itself to "major" pathology of the type encountered in the hospital. The voluntary refusal to become acquainted with this disease is more insidious, because the doctors concerned have heard about this ailment and are aware of certain symptoms, but do not consider them important. Their thinking is that it concerns a general functional pathology quickly baptized "neuro-vegetative" for which there is no treatment and which in any case does not appear to be really serious.

Themselves ignorant of its importance, they deny its existence to those who consult them, and so deprive them of the recognition of the reality of their condition, and the simple and efficient therapies which are available.

At times a diagnosis of spasmophilia is made to reassure the patients and make their symptoms appear ordinary, but it isn't confirmed by complementary examinations, and no therapeutical steps are taken. The patient is thus left to extricate himself from his anguish without assistance, explanations or information ; the spasmophilia then takes on the appearance of being a defect.

The most important role of the physician in this case, as in all others, is therefore, to keep himself informed, to bring his knowledge up to date, to struggle against conventional ideas and stereotyped thinking. He also has a role during the consultation to inform and explain to his patients. This role cannot be reduced to technical gestures, but must truly establish a therapeutical relationship between them.

The medical doctor, aware of this disease, should recognize it in his patient, prove it by clinical examination and diagnostic investigations, detect possible associated pathological conditions, and eliminate other organic ailments, for if thinking of spasmophilia is indispensable, merely thinking of it is in itself unacceptable.

The clinical examination, as always in medicine, starts with an interview (the medical interrogation) which, in addition to symptoms evoked by the patients which cause them to come for a consultation, will allow other symptoms to be detected among those already described, and whose association is characteristic, symptoms that the patient had forgotten or considered not worth while mentioning. This interrogation attempts also to determine the date when the troubles first appeared, the existence or otherwise of several evolving surges, the notion of family antecedents, and possible seasonal recurrences. This interrogation will above all focus on trigger factors which, as we have seen, are always to be found; the trigger being the physical and psychic stress that has thrown this patient off balance, and given and provoked a surge of symptoms that induce him to seek a consultation.

These trigger factors may be obvious (mourning, losing a job, etc.) but sometimes   call for a careful interrogation if they have been forgotten or not understood by the patient. Thus a reducing diet, the ingestion of certain medicines, or simply changes at work, can be difficult to detect: Identifying these factors calls for the flair of a detective, but it is rare for them to go undetected. I insist on the great care needed for such an inquiry and also the discovery of the date when the disturbances started. Although patients are often conscious of a sudden change in their behavior, they may not be aware of the reasons triggering such a change.

The clinical examination itself detects the objective symptoms of neuromuscular over-stimulation:

The Chvostek sign, which is a contraction of the median part of the upper lip (orbicular of the upper lip) after percussion of the cheek in the middle of a line going from the ear lobule to the corner of the lips, the lips being parted

Some other clinical signs of minor interest include :

- The Trousseau sign (appearance of the "midwife hand" after applying a venous tourniquet for ten minutes).

- The Weiss sign (contraction of the eyelid after percussion of the orbitral ridge (apophysis)

- The Lust sign (dorsiflexion of the foot after percussion of the exterior popliteal (knee) sciatic nerve at the head of the splint bone).

On the contrary, the existence of cardiovascular excitement (tachycardia, etc.,) is often noted as well as the hyper-reflexia of the osteotendinous reflexes.

It is absolutely necessary to examine the feet of these patients because in a statistically significant number of cases, the presence of one sided or bilateral concavity is described, which is a weighty argument in favor of the existence of a constitutional factor in spasmophilia. The examination of the hair, nails and teeth can point to disturbances (numerous decayed teeth, soft nails, brittle hair) in relation to the disturbances of calcium metabolism.

The coexistence of the above symptoms, the precise triggering circumstances, the clinical examination showing the symptoms of neuromuscular overstimulation, and other respects being normal, should lead the physician to have diagnostic electrophysiological and biological investigations made which are essential to confirm the diagnosis.

Among the electrophysiological investigations, the electromyogram represents the best examination to prove the existence of objective symptoms of neuromuscular overstimulation. It is simple without any danger and practically painless, and records and studies the aspects of the neuromuscular activity. It is also a common examination, accepted and reimbursed in the same way as an X-ray or blood analysis.

The examination, as it is usually done, records aspects of the muscular contraction at the level of the hand muscle (the first dorsal interosseous muscle, that is, the muscle on the back of the hand located between the thumb and the index finger). This muscle is regarded as representative of the entire bodily musculature. The recording is made by means of electrodes that are placed either on the surface of the skin (external electrodes) or by a needle that is inserted in the muscle (the Bronk needle). The action potential of the muscle, which is the electrical current produced by the muscle, is amplified and visualized on a TV monitor ; these currents are also recorded on a cinematographic type of film, on photosensitive paper, or on magnetic tape for more detailed study.

The examination is carried out according to a well-defined procedure ; firstly, when there is no muscle contraction, nothing is recorded. Then when a voluntary muscle contraction does is carried out, a tracing is made of the potentials, which are more numerous, if contraction is more pronounced. These phases are the same in all subjects. There are usually no differences between spasmophilics and others, which is the reason why the examination is rendered more sensitive by the use of two techniques:

First the ischemia : by means of a pressure reading instrument placed on the arm at the side of the recording, and which is inflated beyond the rate of the blood pressure, the circulation in the muscle being examined is interrupted for a period of five to ten minutes, which puts this muscle in acidosis by producing lactic acid which is not eliminated because of a lack of oxygen.

After five to ten minutes the armband is released and, in the two to five minutes which follow, spasmophilics may show a spontaneous electrical activity in the muscle, made up of electric currents which are repeated (doublets, triplets, or multiplets). This repetitive activity after the end of the ischemia can last over a minute and is altogether characteristic of spasmophilics, in whom the acidosis factor is predominant. It does not appear in other types of spasmophilics and never appears in those who are not spasmophilic.

The second technique is the hyperventilation : the persons examined are asked to breathe deeply for five minutes. This provokes a gaseous alkalosis which, in spasmophilics, triggers a repetitive muscular activity, likewise in the form of doublets, triplets or multiplets, all this lasting for more than two minutes. The hyperventilation test makes it possible to detect a second type of spasmophilic, in whom the symptoms appear in a state of alkalosis or are increased by alkalosis. The distinction between these two types of spasmophilia has practical consequences on the treatment.

Here also, during the hyperventilation test, a prolonged repetitive activity (more than two minutes) never appears in a subject who is not a spasmophilic.

The electromyogram is an examination having great diagnostic value, for the false positives (positive results in a non-spasmophilic control group) are very rare, if the examination is carried out under strict criteria, and the false negatives (negative examinations in spasmophilics) are likewise very rare if the precaution is taken to suspend the ingestion of certain medications which inhibit the repetitive activity for the two days preceding the examination.

As for the diagnosis, a positive electromyogram suffices to confirm the neuromuscular overstimulation by showing a repetitive pathognomic activity (particular to this disease). It also permits specifying the type as being either acidotic or alkalotic, or both, thereby refining the way the treatment is carried out.

An electromyogram should always be requested if the physician suspects a spasmophilia, and it can even be said that a decompensated spasmophilia is shown up by a positive electromyogram.

On the therapeutic level, the electromyogram allows the effects of the treatment to be followed objectively. This is because electromyograms of spasmophilics are rarely completely normal, and the intensity of the electrical signs clearly diminishes when the spasmophilia is properly treated. A reduction in the frequency of the repetitive activity, may be seen both in its intensity, and in its duration, according to the degree in which the circumstances of their appearance has been modified.

The improvement of the electromyogram is parallel to the clinical improvement and the cure of the symptoms, and permits an objective comparison of such improvement if a comparative examination in the beginning is available.

Other electrophysiological examinations are useful in spasmophilia, in particular the electroencephalogram (E.E.G.). The E.E.G. is a recording of the brain electrical activity. This electrical activity of the brain can be disturbed at given points by certain diseases of the brain, and more or less precise lesions of the brain can thus be detected. There is never a localized brain lesion in spasmophilia, and the spontaneous electroencephalographic tracings are always normal, but as we have seen, headaches, migraine, and vertigo are part of the main symptoms of spasmophilia. The E.E.G. effectively determines if there is no local lesion. A spontaneous E.E.G. tracing of spasmophilics is always normal and permits the elimination of a local cause for a headache, but there are also other methods of making the test more sensitive so that it shows particular signs.

Here also, the E.E.G. recording under hyperventilation (ample and deep breathing) is disturbed in spasmophilics : the basic rhythm of the tracing slows down, going from 8 to 9 cycles per second to 5 to 7 cycles per second, and the brain waves become pointed. These changes are not localized but appear on all the cerebral regions recorded.

These aspects, termed "signs of sensitivity to hyperventilation" are nevertheless not proper to spasmophilia, and can exist generally in metabolical disturbances. They are not pathognomonic to spasmophilia, are different from the repetitive activity of the electromyogram, and have great value in association with other electrophysiological and biological clinical signs.

The electroencephalogram shows other interesting features in the framework of spasmophilia. For example, ailments accompanied by loss of consciousness constitute a frequent symptom of spasmophilia and can sometimes be a ground to fear an attack of epilepsy, but the E.E.G. will show that the characteristic brain waves of epilepsy do not exist in such patients.

The overall analysis of the E.E.G. in spasmophilics, however, while showing a normal basic tracing, free of lesion, often shows up diffused minor disturbances, characteristic of the anxiety from which these patients suffer.

This often concerns improperly executed tracings, the basic rhythm of which is associated with much more rapid rhythms caused by the anxiety. Here too, the E.E.G. permits keeping track of the treatment, and the improvement of the spasmophilia is often indicated by a reduction or a disappearance of the signs of sensitivity to hyperventilation and a reduction of the rapid rhythms of anxiety.

Other electrophysiological explorations show different disturbances in spasmophilics, in particular :

- the electro-nystagmogram (electrical examination of the inner ear) which may show signs of central labyrinthic overstimulation;

- the Achillian reflexogram (measurement of the Achilles tendon reflex), which can be modified, either lengthened or shortened. However, these tests concern non-specific explorations for which there are many other causes of modifications outside of spasmophilia and whose practical importance is therefore altogether minor in the context of what concerns us.

Biological examinations form the third great role of the medical examination of spasmophilics. They are often only slightly disturbed, but are necessary so that the physician can establish the diagnosis and treatment.

The calcemia (calcium level in the blood) is always normal. This point is essential, and also enters into one of the denominations of the disease, "chronic normocalcic tetany". It permits the elimination of the possibility of serious hormonal disturbances, in particular, the lesion of the parathyroid glands.

The level of intracellular calcium (present in the cells and not in the blood) could be particularly reduced however, but this is a dosage that is seldom made in general practice.

We have seen studies made by means of radioactive (CA 45) radiocalcium which show a reduction of calcium exchanged from non-bone tissues. This is most likely due to a disturbance of the membrane permeability or by a disturbance of the systems maintaining the intracellular calcium level.

Magnesemia (magnesium level in the blood) is practically always normal, but the level of intracellular magnesium which is stored in the red blood cell compartment (erythrocyte magnesium) can be reduced.

The biological evaluation also includes blood measurement of the protein, phospate, alkaline phosphatases, and electrolytes (chlorine, potassium, sodium). However, these values are usually found to be within normal limits.

Finally, it is necessary to measure the alkaline reserve, which is a reflection of the acid-base balance in the blood and which varies according to different conditions of alkalosis or acidosis.

In the urine, the biological evaluation includes, above all, the calciuria of 24 hours (quantity of calcium excreted in the urine in 24 hours). This may be found to be elevated, thus showing a loss of calcium in the urine despite a normal blood calcium level.

At the close of this triple investigation; i.e. clinical, electrophysiological, and biological, the diagnosis of spasmophilia can be established and affirmed with certainty.

Before undertaking the treatment, the role of the physician is to explain and dedramatize the spasmophilia. First of all, he should reassure the patient regarding the reality of his problems, because spasmophilics who know their symptoms are real have often encountered skepticism, scorn, or irony with respect to their symptoms from people around them, particularly doctors. Listening to the patient, taking account of his ailments, and giving an explanation, even omitting the mechanism which produces his symptoms, already affords relief to the patient. To be listened to, to feel one is understood and believed, and not to be sent away to join the cohort of imaginary patients, already constitutes a measure of alleviation. To name spasmophilia and not dismiss it as a negligible factor but to consider it as a disease that is known and understood, in itself permits a relief of part of the anguish of these patients.

It is therefore essential that the medical consultation be complete and conscientious. For the same reason it is also necessary that the diagnostic investigations be carried out ; for if the spasmophilic knows that his disease is truly real, then the physician must treat it as a genuine disease, with all the diagnostic possibilities that modern medicine affords.

Spasmophilia is a distressing and trying disease. The anxiety which torments these patients is often disabling and the physician should be responsible for his patient, explaining how a metabolic disease can create symptoms, and how these symptoms are maintained and influence his psychic condition. The physician should explain to his patient what he is doing, why he is doing it, and how the prescribed treatment can act. The patient must not be left alone with his illness, but should be accompanied in the diagnostic and therapeutic procedures.

The physician must know the particular fragility of these patients; the risks of decompensation which lie in wait for them in circumstances which are often quite ordinary in their lives. He has to anticipate these risks as much by the treatment as by the information he gives the spasmophilic about his condition.

# THE TREATMENT OF SPASMOPHILIA

The relative complexity of the mechanisms in spasmophilia, the number of factors which come into play in the production of the illness, its different symptoms and the way these symptoms maintain and perpetuate themselves, explains why several therapeutical patterns have been proposed, depending on which level one wishes to act.

As we have seen, there are cellular factors, metabolic ionic factors, hormonal factors, limbic factors and cortical cerebral factors. One can choose to act on one or other of these factors, on several, or on all, the choice of factors often being appropriate to each physician and reflecting his particular conception of medicine.

I want to point out here that the treatment of spasmophilia should be exclusively a medical treatment, that is, conducted by a physician. There are several reasons against self-medication :

The diagnosis of spasmophilia is a medical diagnosis. Although spasmophilia is very frequent, many other ailments can simulate its symptoms and, even if a spasmophilia is present, it may not be isolated but, on the contrary, might be present together with other pathological conditions. We have often seen spasmophilia as a factor aggravating existing pathological conditions. Spasmophilia itself also often creates truly organic lesions of the receptor organs. These organic macrolesions necessitate a specific treatment that goes beyond the framework of spasmophilia.

All these reasons point out the fact that only a physician can unravel what is spasmophilia from what is not. Only an experienced practitioner can distinguish between what is microlesional functional pathology and macrolesional organic pathology. Even more so it is often necessary to detect what is macrolesional pathology induced by the spasmophilia.

The treatment of spasmophilia is a medical treatment, because medicines, even the most harmless, can be dangerous if taken in inappropriate doses. Also the treatment of spasmophilia is always long and sometimes discouraging. Spasmophilics need time, patience and availability. It is the task of physicians to give them this, to explain the illness to their patients, to treat them, to see them again and again, and to support them.

The treatment of spasmophilia can only be effective in the context of a personal and attentive relationship between physician and patient.

There is no standard treatment of spasmophilia. Each patient is an individual case, and apart from the particular form of his spasmophilia, there is his personality, his symptoms, and his problems. In treating spasmophilia, the physician is fulfilling his true function as opposed to what has often been no more than a technician's function.

Before considering the treatment of chronic spasmophilia in its compensated and decompensated forms, one must speak of an attack of tetany which is a medical emergency.

We have seen that it is a serious attack, with or without loss of consciousness, including violent and painful contractions of the limbs and the torso, and accompanied by accelerated respiration (hyperventilation). The attack provokes extreme anguish and is accompanied by a sensation of imminent death. It is an emergency, not because the attack is dangerous in itself to the life of the patient, but because it occurs in an acute situation, suddenly, often at night.

The necessity to act quickly means that the patient and those close to him often do not have the time to call their regular physician or an emergency medical service, either private or attached to a hospital. It is the dramatic character of the tetany attack which explains why it is regarded as an emergency and not its intrinsic danger.

One should play down the situation to begin with, and calm the patient down. This includes also calming those close to the patient, who are often highly alarmed by the attack. Their anxiety adds to that of the patient, and increases it. Also the patient's breathing should be slowed down because during an attack it is always considerably accelerated; if it cannot be slowed down spontaneously, a gaseous acidosis should be brought about, that is, the patient must breathe in a confined atmosphere, breathing in and out in a plastic bag ; we have seen that a gaseous acidosis displaces calcium which then becomes ionized. Having the patient breathe in a plastic bag often suffices to stop the attack or reduce it.

All this should of course be accompanied by an active concern for the patient, explaining the reasons and the mechanisms of his attack, and particularly in searching for the cause which triggered it off.

However, if this first stage (dedramatization, active concern, respiration in a confined atmosphere) is not sufficient, and if the attack persists or becomes worse, a medical step may prove necessary. Since one must act rapidly, an intravenous injection should be resorted to - often of calcium which has a sedative effect. If the patient is seriously disturbed it often becomes necessary to add a tranquilizer injection into a muscle.

In most cases these measures suffice to calm down the attack of tetany. The physician should nevertheless beware of giving frequent repeat intravenous injections of calcium in an emergency, as this may create a state of dependency in the patient at the slightest indisposition.

When the attack is over and the emergency situation has ceased, the examination of the patient should of course continue. His or her spasmophilia should be diagnosed and possibly other associated pathological conditions, and the full treatment is commenced.

The situation is different where it concerns a patient with an initial attack of tetany that marks the beginning of his illness, or on the contrary, of a tetany attack occurring in a known condition of spasmophilia.

In the case of a first attack, the dramatic situation and anguish are at their maximum for the patient and those around him who do not know what it is all about, and the task of the physician is all the more difficult. Attacks occurring in spasmophilics who are aware of their condition and its symptoms, are often better tolerated and in many instances the patients know how to stop their attacks by controlling their respiration or breathing in a plastic bag.

The treatment of chronic spasmophilia aims to act on the various factors which operate in the mechanism of this disease, to correct the disturbances or the lack of balance which exists, and to break out of the vicious circles that maintain the neuromuscular overstimulation.

The physicians are thus led to make use of various therapeutical agents depending on which points they wish to arrive at in the mechanism of the spasmophilia. They can thus:

a) correct the ionic disturbances ;

b) attempt to act on the permeability of the cellular membrane ;

c) correct the alkaline disturbances by relative hyperventilation ;

d) calm down the anxiety ;

e) reduce the neuromuscular overstimulation, either by various medications or various techniques of muscular tension control ;

f) correct the overall disturbances of the organism.

The multiplicity of the factors on which it is possible to act explains why there is no standard treatment of spasmophilia and why each physician selects whatever methods appear to be best adapted to the patient.

The medical treatment of spasmophilia is carried out within the personal relationship of the physician and the patient, and so there is no point prescribing any therapeutical recipes in respect of this.

In the framework of the information given in this book, it is possible to explain the reasons and aims of each therapeutical step - why one may prescribe this or that medication and the action it has, or why one or another technique may be advisable, and its action, constitute useful information for the spasmophilics, but I am not justified in advising this or that therapy. Therapy is and should remain a domain strictly reserved to the relationship between the physician and his patient. A book can inform and explain, but it cannot treat.

Likewise, I do not wish to oppose here what would be "classic" medicine as against "parallel" medicine. This distinction is fundamentally false. The multiple factors of spasmophilia, and we will see, the various ways to approach them, are all part of the same medicine. Giving preference to one factor or another is a matter of personality or conscience, but not of science. In the case of spasmophilia, almost all the functions of the human being are in play, at the cellular, biochemical, metabolical, neurohormonal, neurophysiological, psychophysiological levels. There is no classical or non-classical procedure to deal with all these functions as a whole. At most there are various doors to enter, but it always concerns the same patient and the same medicine.

I add what may appear as a truism, that the physicians see the spasmophilics when they are ill, that is, when they are under an attack of decompensated spasmophilia.

The physicians are treating a decompensated spasmophilic and it must not be lost sight of that the effect, the purpose of the treatments, consists in returning such patients to a position of equilibrium by correcting their various disturbances and then avoiding a relapse. A compensated spasmophilic is certainly in danger, more fragile, and as we have seen, more exposed to stress, but he is not a patient and does not come for a consultation. Advice for prevention of the spasmophilia, as well as the general rules of hygiene that I will develop later on, are addressed to the compensated spasmophilics.

## THE CORRECTION OF IONIC DISTURBANCES IN SPASMOPHILIA

As we have seen in the outline of the mechanisms of spasmophilia, the existence of ionic disturbances are well known in this disease. These disturbances concern calcium, magnesium and phosporus. Vitamin D intervenes in the carrying of the calcium to the interior of the cell.

Calcium: We have seen that the calcium level in the blood is always normal in spasmophilics, but that there often exists an increased quantity of calcium in the urine (hypercalciuria); in these conditions, since the level of calcium is normal and there is a loss of calcium through the urine, it is now admitted that it is useless to administer large quantities of calcium which will not be retained by the organism; it is only in the case of an attack of tetany that calcium is given intravenously, because of its rapid and sedative effect. These injections should not be repeated. The relative falling into disuse of calcitherapy is also justified by the fact that calcium can be dangerous for the kidneys by causing deposits which may form very awkward calculi.

Although it may appear useless and sometimes dangerous to continually administer calcium in large quantities, it is on the other hand necessary to maintain the calcium store of the organism by prescribing a diet rich in calcium (gruyere and other cheese, milk, yogurt, eggs, dried fruit). Calcium in the organism is stored in the bones and, to maintain a normal blood calcium level, the organism must draw on the calcium in the bones which can thus become demineralized making them more fragile (osteoporosis).

We have seen that, although the level of calcium circulating in the blood is normal, and the calcium level in the cells is reduced, then the calcium must therefore enter the cells and this is the role of vitamin D.

Vitamin D : has been used for a long time for the prevention and treatment of rickets. It is used either in its natural form or under various pharmaceutical forms.

Vitamin D fosters the transfer of calcium into the cell and assures the maintenance of the calcium store at the mitochondrial level. It is usually given orally in very low dosages over a long period (several months), but never continually, for vitamin D, or its pharmacological forms, can also be very dangerous to the kidneys, just as a strong dose would be, if continued for too long a period.

Phosphorus : this also acts on the cellular transfer of calcium. Phosphorus increases the level of calcium in the cells and maintains it in the form of phospate - calcium complexes at the level of the mitochondrial level. The phosphorus reduces the calcium loss,    which can be verified by the reduction in the calciuria. Phosphorus is prescribed orally in tablet form and the dose is 1 to 2 grams per day for several months.

Magnesium: we have seen that one can sometimes verify if the level of intracellular magnesium has dropped in spasmophilics. In the case of magnesium, the stock in the organism is reduced (21 to 28 grams, distributed half in the bones, half in the muscles, soft tissues and the blood) whereas the calcium stock is considerable (1500 grams), and it is admitted that there are deficiencies of magnesium in spasmophilics and also that the food ration is deficient in magnesium. In addition, in spasmophilics the magnesium penetrates with difficulty into the interior of the cells, and has a tendency not to be retained there. Here also the role of vitamin D is to facilitate the cellular penetration and retention of the magnesium. Nevertheless phosphorus and magnesium should not be taken together for the two bodies combine to form magnesium phosphate which is, in part, not soluble in the intestines. Magnesium is prescribed orally in the form of magnesium salts (lactate, sulfate, chloride, citrate....) usually in doses of 200 milligrams per day for a period of six months to two years. Magnesium is absolutely not toxic and does not usually present any danger for the organism.

The existence of a magnesium deficiency which has to be corrected in spasmophilics allows us to approach the important question of magnesotherapy. The deficit in magnesium is considered by certain authors as explaining all the manifestations of spasmophilia. Spasmophilia would then be "the typical neuromuscular form of the primary magnesium deficit". This conception may effectively explain certain of the symptoms of spasmophilia, in particular, the neuromuscular manifestations, but we have seen that other mechanisms most likely enter into play.

The accent placed on the primary magnesium deficit explains the importance of magnesotherapy in the treatment of spasmophilia. This deficit, in three quarters of the cases, relates to an insufficiency of intake. Our food ration would be too poor in magnesium; we absorb per day in food only 3 to 5 milligrams of magnesium per kilo; thus amounting to 150 to 300 milligrams of magnesium per day (depending on body weight); it is clear that for the magnesium level to be in equilibrium, that is, that the intake compensates for the losses, a minimum of 6 milligrams of magnesium per kilo per day is needed (from 300 to 450 milligrams for an individual of average weight).

For this reason the treatment of spasmophilia usually includes a daily intake of magnesium salts and a diet rich in magnesium (cocoa, dried fruit, soybean, nuts, dates). However, although magnesotherapy is commonly recognized and prescribed, the explanation of spasmophilia as a primary magnesium deficit does not explain several points. In particular, spasmophilia has a constitutional character, the intake of magnesium is generally the same for all but everyone is not spasmophilic.

It is therefore necessary to bring in the factor of "depletion", that is the constitutional quality of the cellular absorption and excretion of magnesium and of the other ions, and the constitutional variations of the mechanisms for penetration and maintenance of the ions in the cells. At this level, what is important is the permeability of the cellular membrane which may be modified in a specific manner in spasmophilics.

## PROMOTING THE PENETRATION OF CALCIUM AND MAGNESIUM

If it is admitted that the permeability of the cellular membrane plays a role in the genesis of neuromuscular stimulation in spasmophilics, it is tempting to try to act on this permeability. It is clear that this permeability is abnormal; the calcium and magnesium ions have difficulty entering the cells, and having entered, they are not retained. It is difficult to say if the permeability is increased or reduced, but the hypothesis of a disturbance in one direction or another, or in both, is logical. The disturbance is genetic which explains the constitutional and familial character of spasmophilia. Unfortunately it is not known how to act on the genetic disturbance of cellular membrane permeability. On the practical level however, it is known that certain pharmacological forms of vitamin D promote the penetration of calcium and magnesium into the cell and appears to help maintain these ions at the level of the mitochondria.

## CORRECTION OF ALKALINE DISTURBANCES INDUCED BY RELATIVE HYPERPNEA

We have seen how chronic hyperventilation causes symptoms of neuromuscular overstimulation and alkalinize the surrounding environment. Anxiety itself is a factor for hyperventilation which in turn intensifies the anxiety in one of the numerous vicious circles of spasmophilia.

We have likewise seen that Anglo-Saxons doctors regard chronic hyperventilation as the major mechanism in the production of spasmophilic symptoms. It is therefore logical to try to correct the alkaline disturbances and combat chronic hyperventilation.

The techniques of acidification, which aim to combat the alkalinity of the surrounding environment, cannot be pushed beyond certain limits and represents only a palliative treatment.

Gaseous acidosis, it is recalled, is obtained by breathing in a confined atmosphere, for example, into a plastic bag. Metabolic acidosis (at the blood level) can be induced by creating a drain of bicarbonates. Certain diuretics have this action, but they can only be used temporarily.

The correction of chronic hyperventilation is more easily achieved by using certain sedatives, or better yet the patient is told how to breathe and is taught better adapted breathing techniques which entail a slow breathing using the diaphragm, rather than a rapid superficial respiration. The learning of diaphragmatic breathing techniques constitutes a very important reeducation in the therapeutic approach of spasmophilics. We shall also see that the various relaxation techniques should not neglect this aspect.

## CALMING ANXIETY

Anxiety is a major symptom of spasmophilia, and also a symptom which aggravates all the others, which in their turn increase the anxiety. For this reason at the same time that ionic disturbances are corrected and the cause of his symptoms explained to the patient, it could be useful to act directly on the anxiety, at least in the beginning.

There are many medications known as "anti-anxiety agents" which are good for combating this symptom of spasmophilics. This is of course a temporary treatment to break out of the vicious circle, or help the patient to pass through a particularly difficult stage. The anti-anxiety agents alone are never enough but they can be a first approach to the mechanisms of spasmophilia, for they act both at the control level of the mood and emotions and at the peripheral level of muscular tension. Deliberately utilized at particular moments, they can make a valid contribution, even irreplaceable.

## REDUCTION OF NEUROMUSCULAR OVERSTIMULATION

Neuromuscular overstimulation is the key mechanism of spasmophilia and it is central to most of the symptoms. The therapeutic approach to reduce neuromuscular overstimulation can be made several ways: by medication or various medical techniques aiming to produce a reduction of neuromuscular tension, or by employing behavioral techniques directed towards educating or re-educating the control of the spasmophilia on the neuromuscular tension.

The medications of neuromuscular overstimulation are of course, firstly, the medicine to correct the ionic disturbances that we have just seen. This should continue for a long time.

There are also adjuvants which are of substantial interest :

Vitamin. B6 has close relations to magnesium. It forms a combination with amino acids and magnesium which penetrates the cells and it is believed reinforces the action of the magnesium.

The medications called "beta-blockers" act directly on neuromuscular stimulation and suppress the repetitive activity of the peripheral neuron by blocking the system producing adrenalin. They can be very useful to combat attacks of tachycardia or extra-systoles as well as the attacks of contractions in the hands and feet.

The sympatholytics (medication which acts against the sympathetic system) also directly affect the production of adrenalin and can be useful temporarily.

Various medical techniques aim to reduce muscular tension. Acupuncture heads the list of these techniques acting unquestionably on spasm and muscle contraction. Without going into the philosophical, cosmogonic, even esoteric implications of the Chinese theory of acupuncture, it is undeniable that an "occidental" acupuncture exists which by its own techniques, obtains excellent results in the treatment of muscular contractions and the pain that results from them.

We know that in spasmophilics the neuromuscular over-stimulation causes many contractions in the skeletal muscles, including a stiff neck, lumbago, sciatica, lombalgias, etc. It is understandable that the acupuncturist who makes use of efficient techniques against pain can break down certain of the vicious circles of spasmophilia by treating the symptoms which concern the patient. Here too there is a temporary relief, for the vicious circle is ready to close itself again if the full treatment is not followed through.

The mechanism of spinal manipulations which acts by localized stretching of muscular segments can, without doubt, be understood in a similar way as that of acupuncture. Acupuncture of the ear (auricular therapy) establishes a precise correspondence with each organ in the ear, and seems also to have clear-cut results preventing contractions.

Various behavioral techniques aim to educate and re-educate the control of the spasmophilic in respect of his neuromuscular tension since the neuromuscular overstimulation is a problem of nerves relating to the cortico-thalamo-hypophyseal circuit ; it is also logical to think that an individual could manage directly to control his neuromuscular tension.

Relaxation covers several behavioral therapies from the most simplistic to the most elaborate. All the methods make use of bodily experience in support of the therapeutical action. The relaxation techniques aim to obtain a better tension and emotional control (of muscular tension).

There is no point here in describing the various relaxation techniques, but the results are often satisfactory on the psychotherapeutic level well as on the level of symptom control. Spasmophilics can thus learn to relax, to modify their breathing, to learn about their body and its manifestations, and therefore to fight against the anguish of the unknown. The necessity and usefulness of relaxing is generally acknowledged in the treatment of spasmophilia, but the techniques utilized are particularly efficient if they aim at raising awareness of the body. Certain techniques place emphasis on the psychotherapeutic and relational aspect of relaxation, on the emotion of relating with others whether this is real or a fantasy. An excessive resort to psychology in medical relaxation appears improper. The psychotherapeutic relationship is more appropriate between the patient and his physician than with the technician teaching relaxation. The technician acts as an extension of the medical act; it is a prescription by an intermediary and not a way to unload the problems of the spasmophilic on a third party.

Biofeedback appears to be a behavioral technique with a future, in its approach to enable the spasmophilic to control his neuromuscular tension. It is based on learning the voluntary cerebral and psychic control of the psychological functions and the automatic activities such as muscular tension, perspiration, skin temperature, blood pressure, cardiac rhythm.

This method has the merit of not introducing a third party into the physician-patient relation, and in addition, under medical control, the patient guides his treatment and does not undergo it. Technically the procedure is simple; certain physiological activities of the organism (muscular tension, cardiac rhythm, cerebral activity) are collected by means of electrodes placed on the skin which transmit to an apparatus which records this activity and displays it on a screen directly visible, along with sound signals that can be heard by the patient. The patient thus sees and hears various parameters and learns the relation between the psychic and organic functions. The patient who thus perceives, for example, his muscular tension, can then learn to control and master it. He can follow his progress on the apparatus. This relates to learning to recognize the conditions of relaxation and tension.

The procedure entails about 12 to 16 sessions each lasting from 20 to 30 minutes. It is relatively short and seems promising for spasmophilia and also for stress in general.

The main parameters of muscular tension, cardiac rhythm and brain activity are recorded and followed by an electromyogram, an electrocardiogram and an electroencephalogram. The control by electromyogram is done by external electrodes placed level with the forehead muscles. A sight and sound signal is recorded and transmitted to the apparatus. The muscular activity is directly visible, audible, and measurable, by a reading on a dial and by conversion to light and sound signals. The muscular tension can therefore be controlled, and reduced. The reduction of muscular tension reduces the psychological tension and the anxiety. The patient himself controls the learning procedure and the progress of his muscular activity. There is, moreover, a phenomenon of transfer of voluntary muscular relaxation (striated muscles) to the relaxation of the internal organ muscles (smooth muscles) if the muscular relaxation is deep.

Muscular biofeedback can be associated with the biofeedback of skin temperature and perspiration, and by similar techniques the subject can learn to control his skin temperature and perspiration.

Control of the cerebral activity is done by the control of brain waves. Technically, this is a recording of the brain activity by means of external electrodes. This activity can also be visualized. It is known that the presence of abundant alpha waves ( 8 to 10 cycles per second) corresponds to a state of relaxation, whereas rapid waves or beta waves (13 to 30 cycles per second) appear in states of concentration, anxiety and apprehension. Learning consists in increasing the presence of alpha waves and reducing or suppressing the presence of beta waves. The patient must become aware of the link between his state of psychological tension and the aspect of the encéphalographic tracing. The patient must learn to "let go" to obtain the electric and psychological improvement. The recording of the electrocardiogram (also by means of external electrodes) enables a visualization of the cardiac rhythm, its possible rapidity (tachycardia) or irregularities (extra systoles). During the treatment the patient can visualize and follow the slowing down of this cardiac rhythm.

The techniques of biofeedback can be used for all symptoms of spasmophilia, in particular, anxiety, headaches and fatigue.

## TOTAL TREATMENT OF TERRAIN DISTURBANCES

More unified conceptions of medicine do not limit the metabolic disturbances of spasmophilia to the ionic disorders described above. The treatments employed aim at curing the "terrain" in general. This is what homeopathy and the medications of trace elements propose.

Homeopathy is concerned, not with a particular illness but with functional symptoms and the constitution. It is based on the principle that agents likely to do the constitution harm are capable of curing it by infinitesimal doses. Without going into the theory of homeopathy and its therapeutical modalities, it is nevertheless clear that it is, first and foremost a mode of clinical approach. By assuming that a disease is composed only of its symptoms, it leads, before undertaking the treatment, to a study in depth of the situations and a biological evaluation designed to avoid all surprises. The action of the substances utilized is based, not on a theory, but on an empirical comparison of the resemblance of their actions with the psychological singularities of each patient.

It is understandable therefore that this medicine of the person is efficient in spasmophilics, and without prejudging the real action of the substances prescribed, the knowledge in depth of the personality and constitution of the patient is already a therapeutical attitude in itself.

The attitude in homeopathy is, above all, a psychosomatic attitude, which has led to the accusation that homeopathy acts by suggestion or by placebo effect. It is also known that "the medication is the physician," and in this sense, the importance of the functional disturbances induced in spasmophilia makes the appreciable therapeutical success understandable.

Treatments by trace elements propose a medication of the terrain, and assume that a certain number of metals or metalloids (zinc, copper, manganese, lithium, silver, etc.) are absolutely necessary for the organism to carry out certain chemical reactions.

Trace elements that are lacking in the organism must be supplied in very low doses (but nevertheless stronger than those used in homeopathy) and are generally prescribed in ampoules to be absorbed per-lingual. Physicians who use these trace elements have applied themselves to describing a certain number of "terrains" in patients, each calling for specific contributions. Here also a very attentive clinical approach is absolutely necessary to specify the modalities of the symptoms felt. At the doses generally utilized the trace elements never endanger the organism and that is a very appreciable advantage. Depending on the terrain, the specialists in these treatments describe numerous associations which are effective in different symptoms of spasmophilia. For example, manganese-cobalt acts on the spasms and thoracic pains; zinc-nickel-cobalt on fatigue, copper-gold-silver on depressive states, etc. Here too the psychochemical bases of the trace-element action are still blurred, but in any case the attitude of these practitioners is very often benefit to spasmophilics.

To conclude this relatively brief overview of the various therapeutic modalities of spasmophilia, we return to what should be the attitude of the doctor in charge. It is an attitude of broadmindedness and comprehension, also of psychotherapy in the medical sense of the term, that is the support of the patient. The physician treats and in addition explains the disease and its symptoms. The physician plays down and reassures. He accompanies the patient in his illness. The physician does not forget the experience of medical science; he should not lose sight of macrolesional organic attacks, whether they coexist with a spasmophilia or are masked. He must certainly be imbued by the existence of microlesional functional pathology of which spasmophilia is the most striking, but all other pathology must be kept in mind. And, to paraphrase Hélène Michel-Wolfromm, one must be a meticulous doctor before taking on spasmophilia.

# PREVENTION OF SPASMOPHILIA
# AND THE LIFE HYGIENE OF SPASMOPHILICS

The problems of life hygiene of spasmophilics is closely linked to those presented by the prevention of this disease. There are differences in the prophylactic measures to be taken during pregnancy, the treatment useful for infants and young children, the simple dietetic rules which can palliate the various food deficiencies, and finally the precautions, more along the lines of life hygiene, which serve to avoid the decompensation of a latent spasmophilia. One can hardly hope to act on the constitutional and genetic factors of spasmophilia, in particular, on the primary disturbance of the cellular membrane permeability; however an effort can be made to correct the metabolic deficiencies which maintain a large part of the symptoms.

The prevention of spasmophilia starts during pregnancy : pregnant women need more magnesium, at least double the usual quantity for the organism. We have already seen that spasmophilia often causes minor disturbances in pregnancy: insomnia, fatigue, painful uterine contractions, vomiting. A deficit in magnesium which was already present in the mother will be considerably increased during gestation and likewise affect the child who will be born with a very insufficient stock of magnesium. A supplementary supply of magnesium during pregnancy is therefore absolutely necessary. This contribution in mild cases takes the form of a diet rich in magnesium, but in the most serious cases, it is necessary to take a supplementary medicinal supply throughout the entire pregnancy. The condition of the fetus, and afterwards the newborn child, will reflect that of the mother; a deficit can be the cause of small stature or low weight at birth. The additional supply of magnesium avoids forms of spasmophilia of newborns which are truly precocious, temporary or chronic tetany.

The prevention of spasmophilia during pregnancy avoids the giving of birth to spasmophilic children whose character is often difficult and who have numerous problems while growing up.

The supply of magnesium during pregnancy and after confinement also considerably reduces the frequency of post-natal -depression. Many reasons have been put forward to explain the numerous cases of depressive states which occur in the weeks following confinement: psychological reasons, disturbance of the daily life and the relationship of the couple, fatigue...

It appears likely that the decompensation of a latent spasmophilia could well be the responsible determining factor, and gives added value to the preventive magnesotherapy for pregnant women. A balanced nourishment, rich in mineral salts, in particular, magnesium, calcium, phosphorus, is absolutely necessary in infants and young children.. Since the beginning of the century vitamin D {anti-rickets vitamin) has been widely prescribed systematically as fish-liver oil (in particular cod liver oil). It is now given in various medicinal preparations, but apparently less abundantly and less systematically.

It is probable that this relative disinterest in vitamin D therapy on the part of physicians is in part responsible for the recrudescence of cases of spasmophilia that is presently observed particularly in children. Rickets has practically disappeared in developed countries, a return to the systematic prescription of vitamin D in efficient doses, is imperative for preventative reasons. This simple precaution, by itself, would notably reduce the number of nervous, "restless", anxious, children, subject to character disturbances, or who do badly in school although they do not lack intellectual ability. The numerous deficiencies in the diet of mineral salts, in particular, magnesium, calcium, and phosphorus, must not go unrecognized. There are many reasons for these deficiencies in the world today:

- The utilization of nitrogenous fertilizers, rich in potassium, impoverishes plant products of magnesium and calcium.

- Drinking water is frequently softened which reduces its concentration of mineral salts.

- The cereals used in food are deprived of their covering which is the part which most contains the mineral elements and vitamins.

- Sugar and salt are more and more refined which tends to eliminate all trace of magnesium.

- The consumption of dried fruit and vegetables is dropping; these are foods with the highest mineral salts contents, in particular, magnesium and phosphorus.

- The food supply is rich in saturated fats and cholesterol; likewise an excessive consumption of alcohol increases the ionic needs of the organism.

The simple dietetic rules for spasmophilics, are derived from these facts, namely the foodstuffs which can be recommended to ensure a sufficient supply of mineral salts :

- drink mineral water (after having verified the content in mineral salts on its label) and drink it in large quantities: a liter to a liter and a half per day;

- food rich in calcium: cheese, dairy produce (see appendix 3).

- food rich in magnesium: dried vegetables, dried fruit, whole grain cereals, oleaginous food, chocolate (see appendix 4).

- food rich in phosphorus: dried vegetables, dried fruit, fish (see appendix 5)

- reduce or eliminate alcohol which increases the needs for mineral salts. Furthermore, it is necessary to forbid stimulants of the nervous system which favor neuromuscular stimulation, especially coffee.

Finally, the sun has a beneficial effect on the production of the vitamin D in the organism. Exposure to the sun which of course must not be excessive, is good for spasmophilics and helps them to attain their equilibrium.

The correction of mineral and vitamin deficiencies constitutes the first step in the prevention of spasmophilia. The second step comprises measures which aim to reduce or eliminate the trigger factors, which means to learn how to fight against stress factors. The incapacity to face up to, or a low resistance to stress, decompensates spasmophilics; the prevention will consist of increasing the resistance to stress by modifying behavior and the attitude toward life.

Most of the factors of stress are part of life ; to submit to no stress at all is to be dead ! Spasmophilics can be taught how to resist stress. This teaching of resistance to stress, associated of course, with anti-spasmophilic dieting which has just been outlined, calls for modifications of modes of reaction and a change in habits and harmful behavior. It is above all a personal effort of psychological adaptation of the individual to the daily constraints and tensions, complemented by simple methods of relaxation, As we have seen, although the medical relaxation and techniques of biofeedback are made use of in the treatments of decompensated spasmophilia, there are also simpler forms of learning physical and psychological relaxation that can be used daily for prevention.

Relaxing through gymnastics favors a better body expression by knowledge of the body. Spasmophilics must strive to have a relaxed and flexible posture which eliminates faulty positions and ungraceful gestures. The voluntary and flexible movements allow a stretching of the muscles which favors relaxation. The relaxation exercises can be practiced at all times for a few minutes. The tension of the face at the level of the forehead, the eyelids, the jaw, can be attenuated by exercises involving voluntary yawning, and are recommended particularly for people who do a lot of speaking. For stressful situations, the psychological state and physiological tensions are closely linked, the modifications of these physiological tensions acting retroactively on the psychic manifestations.

The purpose of these exercises is to short-circuit the stress by perceiving all muscular tension at its origin so as to reduce it at once. At any moment of tension or anxiety a brief exercise of concentration allows a rapid relaxation. (Refer to appendix 7 for the description of gymnastic exercises for relaxation). Yoga is likewise allied to gymnastic relaxation by an ensemble of postures associated with respiratory exercises bearing on ventral breathing. The practice of yoga is useful as a preventive but insufficient for decompensated spasmophilia.

Sporting activity also permits the "recovery" of one's body. The focus on psycho-emotional tensions is diverted by purely physical stimulations. Sports act as an antidote to psychological stress. They must be practiced in an aerated environment and call for a regular and moderate effort. The sporting activities recommended call for a steady rhythm (walking, cycling, jogging) and will be practiced without attempting to exceed the physical capabilities of the subject. The ideal is to free oneself of the day's stress by doing 15 to 30 minutes of physical activity per day. (see appendix 6 for the sports recommended and those not recommended for spasmophilics). Finally, spasmophilics can adapt their psychological attitude to improve the way they face stressful situations.

The ideal type of behavior consists in reacting with calm, prudence and optimism by emphasizing the positive side of things. A vivid image of explaining what is optimistic behavior with respect to pessimistic behavior is to say that a "bottle half empty is a bottle half full". The psychological profile of a given subject cannot of course be fundamentally modified, but certain practical attitudes in facing life contribute to reduce daily tensions; not to inflict on oneself social, familial, or professional obligations, which are constraining or unpleasant; to be prepared for inevitable changes so as to adapt better ; to arrange for oneself compensating situations of relaxation...

Learn too how to give pleasure to oneself and learn how to accept pleasure from others.

# CONCLUSIONS

To conclude this book which does not pretend to be exhaustive but which is intended to lay out the principal data of a daily problem, I propose to recall what every spasmophilic must keep in mind:

1°/ Spasmophilia is an authentic disease which attacks the organism in its entirety, in its physical, psychic and relational aspects.

2°/ To be spasmophilic, from the aspect of one's constitution, is to have a particularly fragile terrain and to undergo permanent metabolic disturbances.

3°/ In morbid spasmophilia, the terrain, metabolic disturbances and stress, the decompensating factor, are all associated.

4°/ When the trigger factors have disappeared, the illness continues by feeding itself.

5°/ Although the frequency of the spasmophilic terrain is without doubt stable in the population, the insufficiencies in nutrition and factors of stress are, however, in constant progression.

6°/ Diagnosing an unrecognized spasmophilia often permits the release of the patient from inextricable pathological situations.

7°/ The psychic symptoms of spasmophilia constitute neither a mental nor an imaginary illness, but are the symptoms of a metabolic disease.

8°/ The treatment of spasmophilia is possible. It calls on reliable methods, efficient and harmless. They should always be practiced.

9°/ The diagnosis and treatment of spasmophilia is a task for a physician because it may be more dangerous for the patients to overlook a serious lesion than to neglect a spasmophilia.

10°/ Simple hygiene and dietetic rules achieve success in preventing a latent spasmophilia developing into a decompensated spasmophilia.

# APPENDICES

1 - Procedure for checking off the principal symptoms of spasmophilia.

| Symptoms | Never | Sometimes | Often |
|---|---|---|---|
| Intense fatigue | | | |
| Fagging out | | | |
| malaise | | | |
| Tingling in extremities | | | |
| Anguish | | | |
| Headaches | | | |
| Migraines | | | |
| Tightened throat | | | |
| Frequent sighs | | | |
| Emotivity | | | |
| Unstable mood | | | |
| Depressed, somber thoughts | | | |
| Loss of memory | | | |
| Fear of crowd | | | |
| Fear of being alone | | | |
| Insomnia | | | |
| Difficulty falling asleep | | | |
| Early waking; unable do go back to sleep; | | | |
| Combined | | | |
| Internal trembling | | | |
| Unable to stand still | | | |
| Points of pain in the heart | | | |
| Palpitations | | | |
| Oppression in the chest | | | |
| Choking sensation | | | |
| Hypertension | | | |
| Brief fainting spells | | | |
| Dizziness | | | |
| Instability in walking | | | |
| Blurred vision | | | |
| Flies before the eyes | | | |
| Humming and whistling in the ears | | | |
| Knot in stomach | | | |
| Gas excessive swallowing of air | | | |

| | | | |
|---|---|---|---|
| Spasmodic colics | | | |
| Anal pruritus | | | |
| Deteriorated dry hair | | | |
| Soft and brittle nails | | | |
| Frequent decayed teeth | | | |
| Muscular cramps | | | |
| Contraction of the jaws | | | |
| Muscular nodules | | | |
| Aching all over | | | |
| Torn muscles | | | |
| Tendonitis | | | |
| Repeated sprains | | | |
| Twitching eyelids | | | |
| Pain in the spinal column | | | |
| cervicalgias | | | |
| dorsalgias | | | |
| lombalgias | | | |
| Pale fingers | | | |
| Asthma | | | |
| Eczema | | | |
| Urticaria | | | |
| Hay fever | | | |
| Quincke oedema | | | |
| Psoriasis | | | |
| | | | |
| Spontaneous abortions | | | |
| Severe premenstrual pain | | | |
| Irregularities in the menstrual cycle | | | |
| Frigidity | | | |
| Loss of sperm | | | |
| Premature ejaculation | | | |

Without overestimating the value of such a self-observation, it is felt that at least ten clear-cut positive symptoms would indicate spasmophilia and should call for a visit to one's physician.

2 - Identification of trigger factors for spasmophilia.

| Trigger factors | Yes | No |
|---|---|---|
| Cranial traumatism | | |
| Traffic accident | | |
| Surgical intervention | | |
| Recent medical illness | | |
| | | |
| Professional overwork | | |
| Extra-professional overwork | | |
| | | |
| Modification of family conditions | | |
| Reduction of sleep | | |
| | | |
| Pregnancy | | |
| Miscarriage | | |
| Confinement | | |
| Breast feeding | | |
| Hysterectomy | | |
| Natural menopause | | |
| Oral contraception (pill) | | |
| Gynecological infections | | |
| | | |
| Medical treatments | | |
| - diuretic | | |
| - laxative | | |
| - slimming diet | | |
| Toxics | | |
| - coffee | | |
| - alcool | | |
| - tobacco | | |
| - drugs | | |

| | | |
|---|---|---|
| Conjugal disputes | | |
| Family disputes | | |
| Professional disputes | | |
| | | |
| Sexual problems | | |
| Mourning | | |
| Financial troubles | | |
| Change in lifestyle | | |
| | | |
| Other factors known to the patient and not cited in this list (specify) | | |

3 - Calcium Content of Food (in milligrams per 100 grams)

| Less than 25mg/100gm | From 25 to 100mg/100gm | More than 100mg/100gm |
|---|---|---|
| Fruit | dried dates | dried figs |
| mushrooms | All vegetables | broccolis |
| white floor | peanuts | endives |
| corn-flakes | walnuts | watercress |
| noodles | whole wheat flour | parsley |
| spaghetti | | |
| rice | whole wheat bread | leeks |
| honey | unrefined sugar | almonds |
| refined sugar (0) | eggs | hazelnuts |
| meat | | chocolate |
| poultry | | cheese (from 500 to 1000mg/100gm |
| delicatessen | | milk |
| fish | | cocoa |

4 - Magnesium Content of Food (in milligrams per 100 grams)

| Less than 25mg/100 gm | From 25 to 100mg/100gm | More than 100mg/100gm |
|---|---|---|
| | | |
| meat | shell fish | dried haricot beans |
| lean fish | crustacea | split peas |
| eggs | oily fish | shrimp |
| milk | spinach | winkles |
| butter | French beans | clams |
| vegetables | white flour | snails |
| fruit | hard cheese | bran |
| | sweetened dried fruit | unpolished rice |
| | bananas | whole wheat bread |
| | | whole wheat flour |
| | | dried fruit |
| | | almonds |
| | | peanuts |
| | | hazelnuts |
| | | walnuts |
| | | cocoa |
| | | chocolate |

5 - Phosphorus Content of Food (in milligrams per 100 grams)

| Less than 25mg/100gm | From 25 to 100mg/100gm | More than 100mg/100gm |
| --- | --- | --- |
| Fresh fruits | bananas | haricot beans |
| refined sugar (0) | dried dates | lentils |
| honey | dried figs | soybean |
| butter | fresh figs | mushrooms |
| oil (0) | green vegetables | almonds |
| | - artichokes | peanuts |
| | - asparagus | hazelnuts |
| | - carrots | walnuts |
| | - celery | whole wheat flour |
| | parsley | whole wheat bread |
| | potatoes | chocolate, cocoa |
| | white flour | cheese |
| | fresh milk | poultry |
| | | fish |
| | | cocoa |

6 - Sports recommended and not recommended for spasmophilics

| Recommended (regular moderate effort) | Not recommended (irregular and violent effort) |
|---|---|
| Walking | Tennis |
| Jogging | Football |
| Swimming | Weight lifting |
| Bicycling | Rugby |
| Golf | Fencing |
| Ski (preferably cross-country; watch out for altitude) | Squash |
| Rhythmic dancing | Automobile sport |
| Sailing | |

## 7 - RELAXATION GYMNASTIC MOVEMENTS

1.    Exercises for stretching - releasing (5 to 10 minutes)

- Lie down comfortably in clothes which are not too tight;
- Bend toes and turn feet, becoming conscious of the tension, then relaxing; - Stretch legs, knees, and thighs, becoming conscious of the tension and relaxing;
- Contract and relax buttocks;
- Contract fingers then relax;
- Contract forearms, arms and shoulders, then relax;
- Contract the abdomen, then the chest, maintain the tension and then relax;
- Contract the lower back, then the upper back, then shoulders and neck, maintain tension, then relax;
- Contract the scalp, make grimaces, maintain tension and relax;
- Contract muscles of entire body, maintain tension and relax;
- Relax and stretch for a few minutes.


2. Breathing exercises (5 minutes)

- Be comfortably seated and be aware of the way you breathe;
- Think only of the breathing rhythm;
- Follow the movements of breathing in and out


3. Exercises for concentration on parts of body.

- Stretch out comfortably on the back, in clothes which are not too tight, eyes closed;
- Tell oneself that one is to relax completely and one will feel rested;
- Concentrate on the feet while relaxed. The feet must be heavy and relaxed;
- Concentrate on the legs, the knees and the thighs, imagining that they are falling through the floor due to their heaviness and relaxed condition;
- Concentrate on the hands, the wrists, the forearms, the arms, and the shoulders, and feel them as heavy and relaxed;
- Concentrate on the abdomen, then the stomach, then the chest; feel the tension disappearing;
- Concentrate on the neck and the throat and relax the facial muscles, dropping the jaw, with the mind thinking of complete relaxation;
- Remain 5 to 10 minutes in a state of complete relaxation with mind empty;
- Get up progressively, taking one's time, stretch and then commence one's activities.

## ABOUT THE AUTHOR

HENRI RUBINSTEIN, M.D. born in 1942, practices medicine in Paris. On the staff for thirty years of the Neurology Clinic of the Salpetriere hospital, he is specialized in the exploration of the nervous system.

He is the author of numerous medical books, published in Paris and translated in several languages.

Among them :

*The Medecine of Pain, Psychosomatic of Laughter, Life without fatigue, Masked Depression, The Medecine of Pain, The Medecine of Happiness, Failing Memory, Invisible Handicaps, Our Body and its Crises.*

He had also published an essay, written with Roland Topor (1938-1997), a famous French artist : *The Equation of Happiness.*

www.ingramcontent.com/pod-product-compliance
Lightning Source LLC
Chambersburg PA
CBHW060357290526
45791CB00002B/541